Forever Fit

Forever Fit

The Easy-to-Follow, Step-by-Step Life Plan to Improve Your Body and Mind

Join nutrition and fitness coach Dr. Rick Kattouf, one of the nation's top ranked multi-sport athletes, on a journey to better health and fitness.

by Richard S. Kattouf II, O.D.

iUniverse, Inc.
New York Lincoln Shanghai

Forever Fit
The Easy-to-Follow, Step-by-Step Life Plan to Improve Your Body and
Mind

iUniverse books may be ordered through booksellers or by contacting:

iUniverse
2021 Pine Lake Road, Suite 100
Lincoln, NE 68512
www.iuniverse.com
1-800-Authors (1-800-288-4677)

ISBN-13: 978-0-595-33945-7 (pbk)
ISBN-13: 978-0-595-67038-3 (cloth)
ISBN-13: 978-0-595-78734-0 (ebk)
ISBN-10: 0-595-33945-X (pbk)
ISBN-10: 0-595-67038-5 (cloth)
ISBN-10: 0-595-78734-7 (ebk)

Printed in the United States of America

Endorsements

"I can honestly say that without Rick's training and nutrition program, I would not have accomplished half of what I have done so far! Remember, if you buy Rick's book or hire him for personal online coaching, give yourself a fair chance, follow his lead, and results will follow…believe me, *it works!*"

—Rick Shreckengost

"Picking up your business card was the healthiest thing I've done for myself (and family) in years!"

—Todd Huna

"I can only describe my experience with Rick as 'life altering.' Rick is a motivator extraordinaire and walking fitness and nutrition encyclopedia!"

—Bob Shaker

"The best part of Rick's training program is his unbelievable knowledge about training and his confidence in your ability to achieve your goal. He is a great motivator and extremely supportive the entire way."

—Lori Zelenak

"Let Rick take all the guesswork out of training and nutrition. Thank you, Rick; without your easy-to-follow nutrition and fitness program, I would have never been able to gain the respect of my fellow athletes!"

—Frank Spano

"This program really boosted my metabolism, which is a natural cause to gain weight as we get into our 30s…and beyond! The results have been amazing. I strongly endorse it to anybody!"

—Jorge Martinez, MD

Contents

Acknowledgments

Thank you to my mother and father for their unconditional love and support. From day one they instilled a tireless work ethic in me. It was this work ethic that prepared me for life and allowed me to succeed both professionally and athletically. Thank you for believing in me and supporting each and every one of my goals and dreams. A son could not ask for a better support group. I love you both very much.

Thank you to my beautiful sister, Dr. Valerie Kattouf, for her love and support. Thank you for always being there for me.

Thank you to a great friend and client, Loren, who has been a walking billboard for TeamKattouf.

Thank you to a great friend and coach, Mike Niederpruem, for taking me to the next level and making me the best athlete possible.

Thank you to Dr. John Clendenin, a great friend, client, and chiropractor, for keeping my injuries to a minimum.

Thank you to Joy Kimpel and Jim Zador at Artcraft Displays for all of their hard work and great ideas on *Forever Fit's* graphics.

Thank you to Dave Gilk Professional Photography and his photo team for their hard work on *Forever Fit's* photos.

Thank you to each and every one of my clients. Your success has made this book possible. All of you helped turn my dreams into reality.

Introduction

Nutrition, fitness, and health have always been hot topics in this country. Individuals are always trying to lose weight. One new "diet" after the next emerges, and, like a duck to water, men and women are going from one unhealthy diet to the next. Sure, many of these individuals are losing weight…temporarily. How many friends and family members do you know who have lost weight but struggle to keep it off? Are you one of these individuals?

This all-too-common scenario needs to be changed. Let's examine the word *diet*. Diets simply set each and every one up for failure and disaster. Why? Because, by definition, a *diet* has both a specific starting and ending point. Each and every time you are presented with a diet, the presenter is telling you, in so many words, that you are going to fail. You have not yet begun, and you already failed! Have you ever heard someone say, "I am going to go on a diet for the rest of my life?" Of course not. A diet is not meant to last forever. It has closure associated with it. People go on diets after the holidays, before vacations, or before to a wedding—not for life. You may know someone or even you yourself may have been victimized by the "diet con artist" (DCA). The DCA manipulates you into thinking that this new diet you try will work, that you will finally lose the weight you have been fighting for years. So, you buy into it and make the plunge.

OK, you begin a diet starting the first of the year. If you are one of those truly focused individuals, you may even begin a fitness program with your new diet. A new you is about to emerge. This is one of the most common New Year's resolutions, right? You must be commended for your stick-to-itiveness because diets and fitness programs are not easy. Diets make you eat foods that you are not accustomed to, cause you often to become famished due to calorie restrictions, make socializing a challenge due to food restrictions, and even cause you to become edgy because of reduced blood sugar. Working out makes muscles that you did not even know you had sore. With all of that taken into consideration, you continue to forge ahead and stick to the diet as prescribed. Your body weight begins to drop; your clothes fit looser; and family and coworkers start to take notice. You feel great. Your new diet is working.

A few months go by; body weight continues to drop. Congratulations, you have lost twenty pounds. Soon you hit a plateau. You are still on your diet, but your goal weight has not been reached. Frustration begins to set in because you are being strict on your diet, but the body weight won't budge. You are working out more, eating less, and your results are stagnant. Now the avalanche begins.

"What if I just go off the diet for a meal or even a day? I deserve it, right? C'mon, I have been so disciplined for the past few months. I can treat myself and indulge. I will get right back on the diet tomorrow." "Real" food begins to find its way into your new diet.

Tomorrow arrives, and you get on the scale. The scale does not lie, and, as sure as the sun will rise in the morning, so will your body weight. You have put on a pound. No big deal, it's only a pound. That one pound turns into five, then ten. Soon you have put back the twenty pounds (and possibly even more) that you worked so hard to take off. Way to go; you've just been conned.

I am here to tell you that this does not have to be your situation. I do not want you to face the DCA ever again. My program has been so successful for the past thirteen years because of its user-friendly nature. I have taken all of the chemistry, biochemistry, and physiology knowledge I gained through eight years of college and made it very practical. I took the complexity of these subjects and simplified it to maximize the benefits of proper nutrition and exercise. As your personal nutrition and fitness coach, I will take the thinking out of this process for you. This is what my clients have enjoyed so much over the years.

Body weight loss does not have to be temporary. Let me show you how to lose body weight and body fat and keep it off. There are no "special" foods, magic pills, or powders. Sure, I will introduce you to a few "energy products" that my clients and I use on a daily basis. These products are great tasting, healthy, and convenient for a busy lifestyle. This is a straightforward, real-life, easy-to-follow nutrition and fitness program. No matter how busy your lifestyle—children, a spouse, a business, a medical practice, or a law practice—this program will fit in.

Every client I have coached that has undertaken a diet prior to my program is to be commended—not for going on the diet, but for having the discipline and willpower to make such drastic dietary and lifestyle changes. As previously discussed, a diet is neither healthy nor fun, but individuals consistently show the drive and desire to undertake such an arduous task. Now, starting today, I want you to bring that same drive, desire, and willpower to the table. Put your energy toward a program that will drastically change your life, both physically and mentally. I want you to be the next *Forever Fit* success story.

I look forward to the opportunity to assist you in reaching each and every one of your nutrition and fitness goals. Proper nutrition and fitness will allow you to achieve more energy, increase your quality of life, and build your self-esteem. Do it for you, and make yourself a happier, more confident, and more energetic individual. If you are happy and confident with yourself, other aspects in your life will be enhanced as well. I wish you the best; enjoy your journey.

Section I:
Getting Started

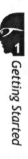

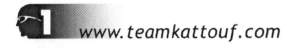

www.teamkattouf.com

Achieving Optimum Fitness

I want to begin by asking you a seemingly simple question: What defines optimum fitness? Definitions will vary from one person to the next, but, when I ask this question of my personal training clients, they frequently cite the following goals:

- Losing weight
- Achieving a certain body fat percentage
- Reducing or eliminating blood pressure or blood sugar medications
- Endurance
- Strength

- Muscularity

- An overall feeling and look

- An enhancement of mind and body

The term *fitness* is very similar to the term *success*. Each of us has a definition of what personal success is. Success comes in a variety of forms. For some it is achieving a childhood dream, such as becoming a teacher, author, or nurse. For others, success may mean the accomplishment of a hard-earned goal, like climbing a mountain or purchasing a first home. Fitness, just like success, has a different definition for each individual.

Although defining fitness is very individualistic, there are a few commonalities. Let's look at the different levels of fitness. Achieving a baseline fitness level is step number one to becoming forever fit. This includes achieving recommended levels of body fat, blood pressure, and blood sugar. Achieving a recommended level of body fat should be your number one focus. Once you start to see a reduction in your body fat, your body weight will reduce as well. As this occurs, you should notice a reduction in your blood pressure and blood sugar.

Body fat percentage is a key factor to which we must all pay attention to achieve optimum fitness (refer to Chapter 3 to read about scales that measure body fat). Through all of my medical studies, it has been shown in research that high amounts of body fat and obesity can lead to cardiovascular disease. Heart disease, high blood pressure, high cholesterol, diabetes, and strokes are more common among those who are obese. It is also important to note that diabetes and high blood pressure are the number one and two leading causes of blindness in the United States. I know some of you may be asking about the role of family history, or genetics, in certain conditions. It is true that heredity and family history do play a role in determining some conditions, such as one's cholesterol levels. Conditions such as high blood pressure and type 2 diabetes, however, are often the result of one's lifestyle.

That having been said, proper nutrition and exercise are the keys to reach a baseline level of fitness. Just as increased levels of body fat can lead to certain ailments, the opposite is true as well. When an individual begins to lose body fat and achieves recommended percentages, the entire body responds in a positive manner. Blood pressure and blood sugar readings soon begin to drop. Cholesterol level readings also reduce. Another great phenomenon that occurs when body fat and body weight begin to drop is an increase in energy levels.

You can now see the whole picture starting to come together. Your body fat and body weight reduce, your medical tests fall within recommended values (your physician is pleased with your results as well), and your energy levels are higher than ever. You look better, you feel better, and your self-esteem and self-image are drastically improved. You are starting to develop the mind and body connection.

A healthy body and mind is a powerful tool for life. Do not underestimate the power of the mind. When you begin to improve your mind, your possibilities are limitless in achieving improved fitness (read the testimonials under Success Stories to see how proper nutrition and fitness drastically improved the body and mind of people just like you). A fit body and mind will lead to an increased quality of life, and I'd bet that you would agree that a high quality of life is extremely important.

During my seven years of private practice, I have examined approximately 6,000 patients each year. Many of these individuals were not anywhere near a baseline level of fitness. They were obese and overly fat, with type 2 diabetes and high blood pressure. They would complain of sore knees, a sore back, and difficulty breathing, and climbing stairs was an effort. These individuals were very angry and frustrated by their poor health and all that comes with it. Their minds and bodies were not fit and therefore their quality of life was quite poor. Their days revolved around visiting one doctor after the next and taking multiple medications. For individuals like this to begin a path to achieve optimum fitness, they must have a desire to change. No one can make you want to change your lifestyle. You have to want it yourself. If you are not at a baseline level of fitness, this should be your fist goal. You *will* be successful because you are reading this book, which means you are ready to make a change!

Once you have reached the recommended levels, especially in terms of body fat, you are now at baseline for achieving optimum fitness. It is now time for you to step back and look in the mirror. What is *your* definition of optimum fitness? Because *you* are reading this in order to reach your own goals of health and well-being, it is important that you consider what *fitness* means to you. You may be completely satisfied with achieving the upper range of the recommended values, or you may be looking to significantly decrease your body fat and get to the lower end of the recommended values. Keep in mind that we are talking about becoming *forever* fit, not fit for three months or six months, but forever. You are about to enter a lifestyle that will assist you in achieving optimum fitness. This is a life plan, *not* a diet. Diets are painful and temporary; a life plan lasts forever.

My goal for you throughout this book is to show you an easy-to-follow, step-by-step approach to help you achieve optimum fitness. Remember, this is a lifestyle change; therefore, patience is the key. I know you want overnight results, but that is unrealistic, not to mention unhealthy. Your excess body fat and body weight did not go on overnight; therefore, it will not come off overnight. I realize that "change" for you may be difficult. Many times in life we choose to take the path of least resistance. In terms of nutrition and fitness, this may mean jumping from one unhealthy fad diet to the next or simply not taking any steps at all to become fit. You become accustomed to fluctuations in your body weight. You tend to procrastinate and say you will start your diet tomorrow, and tomorrow can easily turn into a week, a month, a year, or even a lifetime. I want you to take control of your life and begin to embrace the changes you are about to make. I have made this lifestyle change you are about to undertake very easy to follow. If it were not easy and realistic, I would not have the success I have had with my clients over the past thirteen years.

In no way am I minimizing change. I know how hard change can be, but I also know firsthand the joy that people experience when they make a lifestyle change by following my nutrition and fitness program. As you will see, the nutrition and fitness program I have designed for you is truly easy to follow. The nutrition program is not based on severe calorie restriction. The fitness program does not revolve around excessive hours at the gym. My program is real. You will eat real food for real people just like yourself. The fitness program is designed with your busy schedule in mind.

You are reading this book for a reason, and I commend you for taking the first step in achieving optimum fitness. Be sure to frequently review your definition of optimum fitness. Your mind is powerful, and, if you believe it, you can achieve it. I want you to succeed as much as you do. Congratulations on your willingness to make a lifestyle change! You are now one step closer to becoming forever fit. Think of today as the first day of the rest of your life.

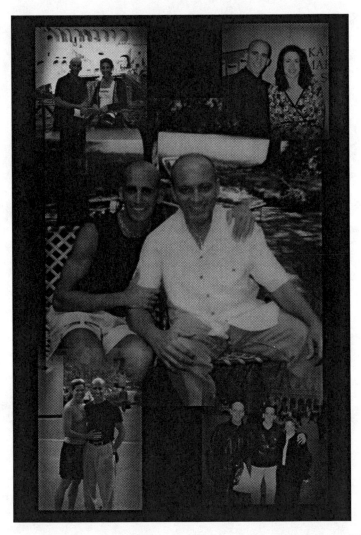

(Top Left) My sister and me in the Colosseum in Rome, Italy. (Top Right) My sister Valerie and me at the Illinois College of Optometry. We are standing in the wing named after my father. (Center) Dad and me hanging out. (Bottom Left) Loren and me in Boulder, Colorado, six weeks after our bike crash. (Bottom Right) Mom, Dad, and me in Belgium.

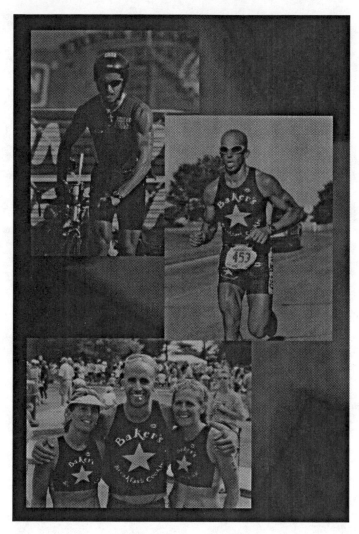

(Top Left) Gearing up for the bike race at the 2002 World Championships in Alpharetta, Georgia. (Upper Middle) Bringing home the victory at an Ohio duathlon. Baker's Breakfast Cookie should be proud. (Bottom Left) Following my victory at an Ohio duathlon, I posed with fellow Baker's athletes. Kathleen Hughes, on my right (from Ohio), is one of the top Ironman triathletes in the country.

Goal/ Dream Setting

"Pursue your dreams with vigor, until fantasy becomes reality!"

As you may have guessed from the title, this is a step-by-step book, and the first step to beginning this nutrition and fitness program is to get into the right mind-set. From this point on you must eliminate all negative thinking. This is what I refer to as "stinkin' thinkin'." Are you one of those individuals that says, "I will never lose weight"? "I have a slow metabolism." "I will never change my body to look like that person!" If this is your mind-set, you must change it now. Thoughts like this preprogram you to fail. Your mind is already in failure mode even before you begin.

I am here to start you on a positive thought process. Our mind is the most powerful part of our body. If we can get control of our mind, our body will follow. You need to reprogram your mind out of the old "stinkin' thinkin'" mode. Positive thoughts will bring positive results. More often than not, people who succeed in their endeavors, whether they be health, business, or social, do so because they maintain a positive attitude, despite any challenges they face. You need to say to yourself, "I will increase my metabolism." "I will lose body weight and body fat." "I will reach a baseline level of fitness." "I will reach each and every one of my goals and dreams." "I will achieve that body I have always wanted." It is the constant repetition of thoughts like these that will bring about positive results. You must believe that you can and will accomplish your goals and dreams, no matter how lofty they may seem.

Each successful client that I have coached has developed a positive mental attitude. The vast majority of my clients did not have this attitude when we first met. They may have been insecure and lacked confidence or self-esteem; some were even depressed. Just as I am teaching you, I taught them how to set their goals and dreams. They learned how their positive thoughts constantly provided them with reinforcement. Soon they developed a strong mind. This strong and healthy minds soon led to healthy bodies. This is a wonderful process to experience. You will soon experience what all of my clients have experienced: increased self-esteem, improved confidence, happiness, and an overall sense of well-being.

Remember the workbooks you used in school (and how much fun was it the first time you found out it was OK to write in them)? Not only did they teach us, but we personalized them by writing our own answers in them. Reaching optimum fitness is hard work, and I hope you'll consider this your own *work*book for personal health. Before you read any further, let's clearly define what you hope to get out of this program. To do so, you'll have to constantly keep your goals in mind. So I ask you, why did you choose to read this book? What is your personal definition of optimum fitness? I want you to take a moment and answer these two questions. Your personal definition of optimum fitness may change over time, and that is perfectly fine. You may find that, as you become fit, you desire a little extra improvement, so feel free to change your personal definition as you begin to embrace the lifestyle changes.

1.   Why did you choose to read this book?

2.　What is your personal definition of optimum fitness?

Next, consider your goals and dreams, which are one and the same. I want you to write down a one-week, one-month, three-month, six-month, and one-year goal-dream. Do not be afraid to dream big. Your goal-dreams may be very similar and relate to the two questions you previously answered. You must be very specific. For example, instead of stating, "I will lose weight," be more specific and state, "I will lose ten pounds of body fat in my first two months and keep it off for the next six months." Take a moment to think about this; what made you read this book? You answered this question in the last paragraph. What is your motivation for wanting to lose weight and improve your fitness? Answering questions like this will help you clearly define your goals.

Aside from your goal-dreams, I also want you to write down two positive statements that will remove your mind from the "stinkin' thinkin'" process. For example, instead of saying, "I just cannot lose weight," say to yourself, "I am ready to make a positive change and achieve optimum fitness. I know that I will achieve my goals by following this program." From this point on, you must believe in yourself and you must believe in the program you are about to embark on.

Just as I mentioned in Chapter 1 that your definition of optimum fitness may change over time as you continue to experience a higher level of fitness, your goal-dreams may change as well. I have coached numerous clients that achieved their goals so quickly that they had to set their bar even higher. They would check off their goal-dreams one by one as they would achieve them. Soon they found themselves reaching their six-month goal-dream in a short three months. It was then time to restructure their goals. I want you to set your mind to achieving your goal-dreams. The excitement you will experience when you reach one of your goals after the next is tremendous. Being able to share this with my clients brings a lot of satisfaction. To hear the joy in their voice or the exhilaration that comes through via e-mail simply reinforces the powerful impact of goal-dream setting and goal-dream achieving. Always remember, if you believe it, you can achieve it! Now jot down those goals and dreams:

- 1 Week:

- 1 Month:

- 3 Months:

- 6 Months:

- 1 Year:

- Positive Thought #1:

- Positive Thought #2:

Good job! This goal-dream–setting process is crucial to make your lifestyle change and your path to optimum fitness easier to follow. Writing down your goal-dreams brings about accountability. You are now accountable to yourself. I also want you to share your goals with someone close to you. Sit down with them and express what your goal-dreams are. Now you are not only accountable to yourself, but you are also accountable to someone close to you. This is exactly why I have all of my clients write down their goal-dreams and share them with me. My clients become accountable to themselves and to me as their coach. It is human nature that once you set a goal, writing it down and then sharing it with others means you will be less likely to stray from your plan. The reason is that you do not want to disappoint yourself or those close to you. It all goes back to accountability. Accountability to yourself and others will breed success. Reading this book will arm you with the necessary tools to achieve optimum fitness and keep you on the path toward becoming forever fit.

By now, everything is beginning to fall into place. You clearly understand why you are reading this book. You have defined what optimum fitness means to you, and you have written down your one-week through one-year goals. You are now ready to begin a great journey. To make this journey as successful as possible for you, I will share two simple words with you that I share with every one of my clients: *have fun*. Keep in mind, a diet is painful, but a life plan should be fun. Continue to repeat these two words to yourself throughout your journey. Soon, having fun with your goals, nutrition, and fitness program will become ingrained in you.

If we have fun in life, we are more likely to be successful. Think back to a successful time in your life when you were having fun. Try to bring these positive feelings you experienced at that time to the surface. I want you to take a moment, close your eyes, and relive this past success in your mind. Bring back those feelings of joy you experienced. Visualize the sequence of events that led to this successful moment. In your mind, try to recreate this time as exact as possible. Do you recall how good you felt at that moment? In your mind, can you see the smile you had on your face? It is this feeling, this attitude, that I want you to have while you are on your path to optimum fitness. If you are having fun, you will succeed. When we are having fun, we are much more relaxed. This causes us to put less unneeded pressure on ourselves. Every time I enter a race, I continually repeat to myself, "Have fun." I know from experience that this relaxed attitude produces a successful outcome. I do not want you to confuse a relaxed attitude with an "I don't care" attitude. You can be relaxed and focused at the same time. I am very focused on my goal-dreams just as you are with yours. Being relaxed and having fun simply allows your mind to be clearer. Just as you did with your goal-dreams, I want you to write down your successful moment and the fun you experienced. The situation you just visualized is what I want you to put into words.

Before you write this down, however, let me share one of my successes with you in case you are having a difficult time mentally recreating yours. When I think back to a time in my life when I was having fun and was successful, I go back to May 1997. My eight years of medical education were finally behind me. I was hours away from my optometry school graduation where I would officially become a doctor. I visualize this day as if it were yesterday. It was a great day in my life that brought me a great amount of joy. I visualize the eight years of hard work that led to this glorious day. The fun that I experienced on this day is the fun I try to recreate in all phases of my life. Whether it is practicing optometry, coaching my clients, training myself, or writing this book, I am always making sure that I am having fun. Just as having fun keeps me relaxed and as productive as possible, this "having fun" attitude will do the same for you. Take a moment and write down your moment. You may have more than one. If so, write down as many as you can. Be very specific in the feelings you experienced at that time. I want you to visualize this situation, write it down, and bring it to life.

Write down one or more successful moments that you experienced in your past. Be sure to recreate the positive emotions you experienced:

Successful moment #1:

Successful moment # 2:

Now that you have written down your goal-dreams, positive thoughts, and successful moments, take a moment to review them. To keep yourself on the path to optimum fitness, I want you to read over your goal-dreams each night before you go to bed and ask yourself, "What did I do today to get one step closer to reaching my goals?" As you lie there in bed, visualize your past successful moment and relive, in your mind, the positive emotions you experienced. This may sound like a lot, but in actuality this will only take you but a minute or two each night. You are only asking for a minute or two from yourself each day to achieve a lifetime of an improved body and mind. This simple process will keep you focused, knowing you are accountable to yourself and others. Congratulations on getting one step closer to achieving optimum fitness. I want you to turn each and every one of your goal-dreams into reality!

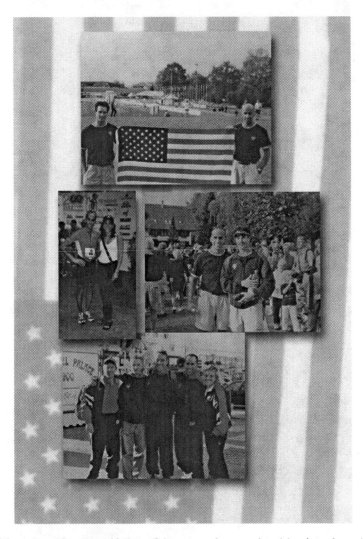

(Top) Jon Hastings (fellow Ohioan and great duathlete) and me in Affoltern, Switzerland, at the 2003 World Championships. (Middle Left) My sister and me in Rimini, Italy, at the 2001 World Championships. (Middle Right) Jon and me again in Switzerland at the Parade of Nations. (Bottom) Heather Gollnick (far right), 3x Ironman Triathlon champion, me, and other members of the 2001 World Championships in Calais, France.

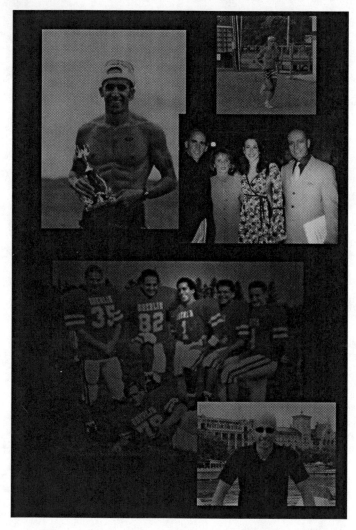

(Top Right) Hometown 5K race on July 4. Check out my stars and stripes shorts. (Top Left) Celebrating my age group victory. I am sporting temporary tattoos of my sponsors. (Middle Right) My mother, father, sister, and me at the Illinois College of Optometry in Chicago. (Bottom Center) Having fun with a few of my Oberlin College football teammates. That is me, #1. How about all that hair? To my right, #82 is Joe Martin, a very good friend of mine while we grew up. Joe is now a cardiologist in Cleveland, Ohio. (Bottom Right) Me hanging out on Lake Zurich in Switzerland during the week of the 2003 Duathlon World Championships.

3 *www.teamkattouf.com*

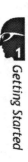

Monitoring Your Progress

There are numerous methods to monitor your progress during your nutrition and fitness program. The scale, obviously, is the easiest and most popular way to monitor. I do feel the scale is important, but other methods are just as important. Do not get too hung up on your body weight. Right now, you are probably saying, "What do you mean 'don't worry about body weight?' That is why I am reading this book." Body fat loss is more important than *just* body weight. The goal is to lose body fat as opposed to losing weight from water loss. By losing body fat, you will find that your progress is not temporary…the weight *will* stay off!

As previously mentioned, your excess body fat and body weight did not appear overnight; therefore, it will not come off overnight. Remember, patience is the key. Becoming forever fit is a life plan, not a temporary fix to your weight gain. Losing water weight, which will happen if you were to adopt a fad diet, is simply temporary weight loss. After someone loses weight following a fad diet, it is all too common for them to put back all of their weight once they stop the diet and begin to eat "normal" once again. This significant amount of weight loss mainly occurs due to the restriction of carbohydrates. When carbohydrates are restricted, the body loses a lot of water. This loss of water translates into body weight loss with minimal to no body fat loss. This is not going to allow you to achieve optimum fitness, thereby not allowing you to become forever fit.

According to skin fold data from the National Health and Nutrition Examination Survey (NHANES II), the following are recommended body fat percentages: 20–35% for women age 34 years or less, 23–38% for women between the ages of 33 and 55, and 25–38% for women over 56 years old. Recommended body fat percentages for men are as follows: 8–22% for men 34 years or less, 10–25% for men between the ages of 35 and 55, and 10–25% for men over 56 years old (*ACSM's Resources for the Personal Trainer*, pp. 86–87). Optimal blood pressure is considered to be less than 120/80, normal blood pressure is 120–129/80–84, and fasting blood glucose should be 60–109 mg/dL (*ACSM's Guidelines for Exercise Testing and Prescription*, sixth edition, pp. 41, 48).

Losing body fat is the key to permanent weight loss. I realize it is difficult to conceptualize that weight loss from body fat compared to weight loss from water. Unfortunately, by today's standards, body weight seems to be the sole focus. There is very little if any information that is available to the general public about the importance of body fat percentage and overall health. There is so much focus on one number…body weight. In my opinion, this is a huge reason why obesity and cardiovascular disease is at an all-time high in the United States. Research shows that a very high percentage of Americans are obese. My concern is that, although this percentage is quite high, it is solely based on one's height versus weight. Height and weight are very misleading factors when determining obesity. Consider these two prime examples. I coached a male client, forty-three years of age. He was 6'2" and weighed 180 pounds. I am sure you would consider this to be an acceptable weight, as would a height and weight chart. A height and weight chart may show a more acceptable weight for this male to be closer to 170 pounds, but would not consider this person obese. When I measured this gentleman's body fat percentage, it was 29.5%. This gentleman is obese by the recommended body fat percentages mentioned earlier. Another example is a forty-two-year-old female client. She was 5'2" and weighed 122 pounds. Once again, a height and weight scale would not consider this woman obese. I measured her body fat at 40.1%! Just like my male client, this woman is obese. As I mentioned earlier, I want to change your thinking. You have done very well so far: you determined why you are reading this book, defined optimum fitness, wrote down your goals and positive thoughts, and visualized previous success. Now I want you to change your mind-set toward and understanding of obesity. Up until now, you thought obesity was obvious. Obesity to you was embodied by person who was extremely large in structure. Please review the two examples I just gave you, and you will realize that obesity goes well beyond body weight. If our researchers would use body fat percentages instead of height and weight scales to determine obesity in the United States, the numbers would be even more astounding. Just as you are in tune to what your body weight is, I want you to start looking at your body fat percentage as your key to success. As you start to see a reduction in your body fat, you will see a subsequent reduction in your body weight. You can expect to lose between .5 and 2.0 pounds of body fat per week. As I learned in my medical studies, you have to burn 3,500 calories each week to lose one pound of body fat.

Let's break this down. Over a seven-day week, this means you would have to burn, on the average, 500 calories more per day than you consume. So, if your total calories burned in a day were 2,500, and you consumed (ate) 2,000 calories, you are right on track. You just burned 500 calories more than you consumed. Now, do not be intimidated by all of these numbers. Keep in mind, I designed an easy-to-follow plan for you; therefore, you will *not* have to count calories. I simply wanted to put weight loss and body fat loss into perspective for you. When you see these reality shows or read about these individuals that lose ten pounds in a week, you can be assured that the majority of this weight loss was water and not body fat. To burn ten pounds of body fat in a week, you would have to burn an additional 35,000 (that equals 5,000 additional calories per day) compared to what you consume!

One of the best purchases you can make is a scale that measures both body weight and body fat percentage. (You can search body fat scales online. Many large department stores and health food stores carry these scales.) You need to get your baseline body weight and body fat (if you have a scale that measures both). The best time to get your body weight is immediately upon awakening after emptying your bladder. The most accurate measurement of body fat on these scales is at night prior to going to sleep. The reason is that upon awakening, dehydration can tend to alter the body fat measurement. In summary, simply be consistent with your body weight and body fat measurements, whether you do it in the morning or at night. This will increase reliability. Try not to measure yourself more than once per week. There are other methods to obtain your body fat percentage. If you belong to a fitness center, you can ask them if they have the means to obtain body fat measurements. Most likely they will use either bioelectrical impedance analysis (BIA) or skinfolds. BIA works by passing a small painless and harmless electric current through the body. Skinfold measurement is obtained with calipers. Three to seven sites on the body are measured to determine your body fat percentage. More sophisticated means include hydrostatic (underwater) weighing. The key is to obtain your body fat percentage with one of the above and continue with the same method each time. You do not want to compare a skinfold measurement to a BIA measurement. For ease of use and good reliability, I recommend purchasing a body fat scale. I have used one for some time, and I am very pleased with it, as are my clients who have one. I have had my body fat measured by skinfold a number of times throughout my life. Just like you, I like convenience; therefore I like the body fat scales.

Aside from weighing yourself and obtaining your body fat percentage, you will want to take baseline body measurements from the following regions. Simply use a tape measure to obtain readings. You may want to have someone help you to ensure accuracy:

1. Neck (Measure the collar of a well-fitting shirt. Lay the collar flat, and measure from the center of the collar button to the far end of opposite buttonhole.):

2. Chest (Measure just under arms and across shoulder blades. Hold the tape level and taut.):

3. Upper arm (Loop tape around widest part of upper arm.):

4. Waist (at level of navel):

5. Hips (Measure around fullest point of hips while standing.):

6.   Upper thigh:

7.   Lower leg (calf):

After you get your baseline readings, repeat these measurements every three weeks. As you begin to lose body fat, you will see a reduction in these measurements.

Photographs are extremely helpful in monitoring your progress. Take a baseline photo of yourself before beginning this program. Men, it is best to wear only shorts. Women should wear a two-piece bathing suit. As with the body measurements, repeat these photographs every three weeks. Make sure you wear the same clothes for each photograph (unless, of course, you have lost so much body fat and your clothes are falling off).

Another great indicator of improved fitness and health is the fit of your clothes. When you begin this program, your body will go through some extreme changes. Notice how your clothes are fitting. Are your pants, shirts, and so forth much looser? Are you able to fit into smaller sizes? I am sure you have clothes in your closet that you would love to fit into. Keep these as a reminder of your target size. True body fat loss can bring about some unique circumstances. Let's say you have a pair of jeans that fit twenty pounds ago, and let's assume that previously you lost this weight on a fad diet (therefore your weight loss was mostly water weight loss). Now that you are on a path to optimum fitness, you begin to lose body fat. It would not be uncommon that after losing ten to fifteen pounds of body fat that you will fit comfortably into those jeans that fit twenty pounds (of water weight) ago. I have seen this occur with all of my clients who followed my nutrition and fitness program.

I have discussed the power of a strong mind and how important it is to think positively. Because body fat is not a common measurement, and you probably have no clue what yours may be, your percentage may surprise you. You very well may go through a lot of emotions, especially if it is extremely high. No matter what your body fat percentage is, I want you to stay calm, take a deep breath, and stay relaxed. If it is high, worrying about it is not going to help.

Do you remember the stinkin' thinkin'? We only have so much mental energy to use; therefore, I do not want you to burn any of this energy in a negative manner. If your body fat shocks you, I want you to turn this negative energy and negative thinking into positive thinking. Use this as another motivating factor to get on your path to optimum fitness so you will become forever fit. Feel free, once you obtain your body fat percentage, to adjust, add, or change some of your short-term goals. If your percentage does not fall within your definition of optimum fitness, set a realistic body fat percentage goal for yourself. There is nothing wrong with wanting to take baby steps. Actually, I highly recommend this.

For example, if your body fat percentage is 45% as a female or 35% as a male, I am sure you want to reduce this percentage. Sure, you want to get to 35% and 25%, respectively. This is a large reduction, especially for a short-term goal; therefore, take baby steps and set your goal at 43% and 33%. This is why I had you record your short-term and long-term goals. You have to crawl before you walk. Achieving these short-term goals is what will keep you focused and allow you to have fun.

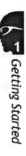

The Balancing Act

Just as my entire nutrition and fitness program is based on balance, bringing your life into balance will bring you increased vitality, long-term health, and inner peace. I commend you for entering this new phase of your life. Your new lifestyle will necessitate change. Change is not easy for the individual engaging in it or for those with whom you surround yourself. It is imperative to have an intimate support group that will encourage you along the way. This support group may be your spouse, boyfriend, girlfriend, children, friends, or family members. I invite you to share your goals and dreams with those in your support group. As I mentioned in Chapter 2, this will not only make you accountable to yourself, but to those close to you as well. Accountability will help pave your path to success. As your progress through *Forever Fit*, share your ups and

23

downs with your support group. This will make your newfound lifestyle that much more fun and enjoyable.

If you are in a relationship, your spouse, boyfriend, or girlfriend will most likely be a major part of your support group. Over the many years of coaching, I have seen many couples that did not show support for each other. By reading this book, you obviously are the one that is ready to make a lifestyle change. I designed this program in a way that will not take away from home and family life. The fitness program is based on a three-days-per-week plan with one optional day. This will bring about success without being too time intensive. The nutrition program is designed for life; therefore, you can enjoy it with your loved ones—something that a fad diet cannot accomplish because of its severe nutrition restrictions. This program, or recipe for success, will not only keep you in balance, but it is itself an act of balance. The recipe keeps your need for fitness discipline balanced with your desire for routine flexibility.

Now that you have clearly defined your goals, you likely want to be able to achieve each and every one. This will require a positive attitude and a desire to have fun. Support from your loved ones will be extremely helpful in this regard. You have already shared your goals with those close to you, and this will keep all of you on the same page. They know what your objectives are, and they will want to see your success as much as you do. Knowing that you have positive support will deepen your sense of accountability, thereby strengthening your desire to achieve optimum fitness. This is the balance you want to achieve—your personal desire to become forever fit and positive support from those close to you. This will keep everything fun, and, when you are having fun, your mind will be clear and strong and you will be able to focus on your fitness goals.

With a small time commitment, you will be able to improve physically and mentally, and to achieve better overall health without disruption of family or work. As you progress through this program, you are going to see many positive physical changes. You will begin to enjoy the training and nutrition and soon begin to realize that the changes you have made were not so difficult. Soon, you begin to crave the training. Your day will not seem complete if you miss a workout. You will become very passionate about your training.

I used the word *passionate* in the previous paragraph in place of the word *obsessed.* Being passionate about training is a good thing. Whether you have been working out for some time or have just begun, you will find that working out "centers" you; the workouts train your body and mind. If you work out first thing in the morning, you will feel you can take on the day with a renewed sense of vigor and energy. If you work out at night, you will find that the training clears your mind and body of life's daily stresses. This allows you to sleep well and wake up to take on a new day and new challenges. This is a passion, not an obsession. This is a very healthy way to live, and this is what will allow you to keep a balance in your life. If you are passionate about your life plan, this will enhance your family life.

Obsessions, on the other hand, will disrupt many phases of your life. I know you want to make a lifestyle change and that you are ready to focus on all of your goals. Your desire to make a change is probably greater now than ever. You have a lot of positive energy that you want to put toward becoming forever fit. I want you to channel this energy into a passion, not an obsession. When you become truly passionate, you will embrace the quest for change you are embarking on, your goals will become clear, and your mind-set will be stronger than ever.

Your passion will be quite visible to your support group. You want to be able to share this passion with your spouse, boyfriend, or girlfriend. As you begin to get more healthy and fit, others will start to take notice. This is great, but many times your loved one begins to resent the added attention you receive. Not only may the added attention create resentment, but the *minimal* time spent away from the home (at the gym) may possibly add to it as well. In order to combat this, try to get your loved one actively involved in your nutrition and fitness program with you. The two of you can work out together, eat the same foods, and enjoy the benefits of a healthy lifestyle together. This is why in Chapter 2 you not only wrote your goals down but shared them with your loved ones. By sharing your goals, you are expressing the changes you desire, and your loved ones will want to share in your passion. Remember, this is a life plan; therefore, both of you can enjoy the highest quality of life together.

I designed *Forever Fit* to be extremely user-friendly. If you are following the program as prescribed, there is no reason that your workout time commitment should disrupt your everyday life. Working out and eating well is a very healthy passion. Obsessions are unhealthy and can disrupt your focus. Passions allow you to be more concentrated and focused. If you are passionate about achieving optimum fitness, you will not only enjoy it but you will embrace all aspects of it. By reading this book you are expressing your readiness for change. Now it is up to you to master the balancing act and to enjoy the success that comes with it.

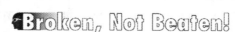

"Life is an obstacle course with me as the primary obstacle; if only I could get out of my own way."

Many times, life can seem cruel. Adversity can rear its ugly head in different forms throughout our lives. Dealing with this adversity can be very challenging. The key is not to let these adverse situations beat you. I want to share my story with you.

As I was writing this book, I suffered a slight physical setback. On May 30, 2004, I was involved in a bicycle crash that left me with a broken collarbone, severe road rash (like a burn), and a severe concussion. My dreams of success in 2004 were crushed in an instant. I was scheduled to race the duathlon world championships in Denmark in August 2004. I could have begun to feel bad for myself, but instead I chose to turn a bad situation into a positive one. I never missed a day of work. I was back in my office, examining patients (in extreme pain I might add). Four days following my accident, I was in the gym, lifting weights with my legs. I refused to let my injuries cause me to lose focus.

Just as you, after reading Chapter 2, I had my goals written down. I had to significantly restructure them due to my circumstances. All of a sudden, my goal of completing my book moved right to the top of my priority list. Before my accident, training and racing in the world championships was very high on my list of goals. It was my goals that kept me focused throughout this injury. This allowed me to turn my longtime dream of writing a book into reality.

I share my story with you because, throughout your journey toward optimum fitness, you will face adversity, just as I have. You must learn to deal with this adversity and do all you can to turn this into a positive source of motivation. This is where you will see the importance of writing down your reasons for reading this book, your definition of optimum fitness, your goals and dreams, your positive thoughts, and your past successful moments. Writing down and reviewing this will keep you focused. I know you want to make this lifestyle change so bad. You are passionate about achieving your goals and dreams. Always keep in mind your accountability to yourself and to others. How will you respond, no matter how minor or major the obstacle may be?

When you come home from work and you have had a very stressful day, you probably want to vent and lash out. You may be the type of person in the past that used eating as a pacifier. Your first reaction may be to binge. You may want to eat everything as though it is your last meal. This is when you need to take a deep breath and try to focus. Remember the big questions and the answers you wrote in Chapter 2. Why are you reading this book? What are your goals and dreams? Are you going to let your daily frustrations lead you off the path toward optimum fitness? This is where you must keep a strong mind and stay on the correct path. Try not to act on your emotions of frustration. You are accountable to yourself and others. Straying away from your path toward optimum fitness will only frustrate you in the end.

As you begin to make your lifestyle changes, you may not find that you are getting results as quickly as you would like. In the past when you tried a diet and this occurred, your first reaction was probably to get frustrated and stop the diet immediately. Since this lifestyle change you are undertaking is not a diet, but a life plan, quitting is not the answer. You are making an investment in yourself for life. You want to achieve optimum fitness and become forever fit. The return on your investment will be an increased quality of life, increased confidence, increased self-esteem, a healthy mind and body, and happiness in all phases of life. Try not to let your frustrations get the best of you in situations like this one. Instead of becoming increasingly frustrated, reassess what you have been doing. Did you write down your goals and dreams? Are you following the nutrition program exactly, or are you binge eating more often than you think? Are you following the exercise program as prescribed or are you making your own modifications?

Some of my most successful clients have found themselves in situations like the ones I just described. They became increasingly frustrated with their lack of progress. If I asked them if they were following my program as prescribed, they would say that they were. But when I reviewed their program with them, I found numerous areas that they were modifying themselves. I showed them how to fix their issues and they were then on their path to optimum fitness. These were clients that were ready to quit on themselves and quit on me. Once they were able to get back to a proper mind-set, they were able to refocus, review their goals, and return to the path toward optimum fitness.

Let's say you are really enjoying your lifestyle change and you are reaching your goals one by one. You are happier and more confident than ever. You never thought you could feel or look as good as you do. All of a sudden you have a minor physical setback such as a minor surgery. Your doctor tells you that you cannot work out for two weeks. You are crushed! Your workouts were going so well and your body fat and body weight have been consistently moving in the right direction. You immediately think to your past when you would stop a diet and exercise program and your weight went right back on. Once again, you feel this will happen. After the initial shock, you begin to think about your goals and all the hard work and commitment you have been putting into your life plan. All of a sudden you hear the words you just spoke...*life plan.* You realize once again that you are in this for life. Just because you cannot work out does not mean you will regain the weight you lost. Not being able to work out does not mean you cannot continue to eat well. At a time like this, if you focus on your nutrition, you will keep your weight off.

Over the years I have had a lot of individuals express their weight gain issues with me. As a nutrition and fitness coach, I have found that people just want to share their story with you whether it is good or bad. I have talked to so many people that would blame their weight gain on a similar scenario that I just described. In no way am I minimizing the inability to work out due to similar circumstances. When these people are honest with me, they also begin to tell me that their nutrition was worse than ever during this time. They became depressed and this led to excessive eating. I know you will not let this happen to yourself, just as my clients do not let this occur. The first four chapters have showed you how focusing on your goals and dreams, being accountable to yourself and others, having a support group, and keeping a balance in your life will allow you to better deal with life's stresses.

Life will throw us all curveballs. With this brings us many unwanted stresses. We cannot eliminate the stress and adversity, but we can learn how to manage it more effectively. Throughout this nutrition and fitness program you are about to engage in, you will experience many ups and downs. Family, work, and other obligations will bring unwanted stress into your life. During these times I want you to stay positive and focused. Reiterate your goals to yourself so as not to lose perspective, and as I have dealt with life's stresses, you too may become broken…*not* beaten!

Section II:
Nutrition

Achieving Optimum Nutrition... Understanding Carbohydrates, Proteins, and Fats

There are three very important factors to achieving optimum fitness. These include proper nutrition, weight training, and cardiovascular training. When you balance these three factors in your life, you will achieve positive results. And when any of these factors are compromised, the results will obviously be compromised.

Over the last thirteen years, I have trained numerous individuals. I have worked with men and women of all different body types, goal-dreams, and so forth. I have observed a few common trends:

1. A majority of those that I have worked with were overweight not due to excess food intake, but an insufficient caloric intake.

2. Faced with the prospect of losing weight and increasing health and muscle development, most individuals are eager and motivated to start and continue a fitness program.

3. Most individuals have a difficult time conquering their poor nutrition habits.

I will show you an easy and successful method to establishing a good nutrition and fitness program. This nutrition program is a life plan. It includes real food for real people just like you.

Carbohydrates

Carbohydrates are the cornerstone of your nutrition program. They are critical for providing your body with the fuel it needs. Many of you may have tried a low-carb diet in the past. Yes, these low-carbohydrate programs will provide weight loss…a *temporary* weight loss! Let's examine why a low-carb program promotes rapid weight loss.

Carbohydrates are "water loving" macronutrients. Therefore, when carbohydrates are ingested, your body will retain a certain amount of water. If you significantly cut your carbohydrate intake, you will lose a lot of water. This water loss is what translates into the body weight loss experienced on low-carb programs. The key to a good quality nutrition and fitness program is not body weight loss, but body fat loss. Slashing your carbohydrate intake does not promote body fat loss. When body fat is reduced, the body weight will stay off, but when water is lost, the body weight will go right back on…and then some.

Throughout my many years of studying biochemistry and human physiology, I have learned that slashing your carbohydrate intake and increasing your protein intake could potentially lead to a number of physiological effects. First of all, your brain needs fuel to function. The primary fuel source for your brain is glucose. Glucose comes from carbohydrates. By eliminating or significantly reducing your carbohydrate intake, you can start to feel light-headed, dizzy, and an overall lack of energy. When carbohydrates are ingested, they will get converted into a substance called glycogen, which is stored in your muscles. Think of your body as a car and the glycogen as your fuel. If your car runs out of fuel, it will not run. The same holds true for your body. If you run out of glycogen, you will not have the fuel to keep going. Reducing your carbohydrate intake will lead to low glycogen levels. This is as if your body is operating on empty. This is why fatigue and a lack of energy will begin to set in.

Due to a lot of misinformation available to the general public, many individuals have become to believe that carbohydrates are not good for you. Just as I have taught you to change your mind-set earlier in this book, I want you to change your mind-set in how you view carbohydrates. Carbohydrates are not your enemy. They are good quality fuel for your mind and body. This is a life plan for an improved body and mind. Feeding your system with the proper macronutrients will lead you to optimum fitness. Any macronutrient (carbohydrates, proteins, and fats) eaten in excess will create unwelcome circumstances. Just as Chapter 4 talked about the balancing act in your life, I have designed your nutrition program around balance. I want you to believe that carbohydrates are not just OK to eat, but essential. If you come from a low-carb lifestyle, I realize this change of thinking can be difficult.

As a nutrition and fitness coach, educating clients about the necessity of carbohydrates has been my biggest challenge over the last few years. Numerous clients have hired me that have come from a low-carb lifestyle. Obviously this lifestyle was not the answer for them and this is why they hired me to coach them. The challenge for me has become to change their thought process. I teach them and educate them on the importance of carbohydrates. Once they begin to see their goal-dreams become reality, they soon become believers that carbohydrates are not the enemy as they were previously programmed to think.

Foods that contain good quality carbohydrates come in numerous varieties, such as fruits, vegetables, oatmeal, wheat bread, brown rice, pasta, potatoes, energy bars such as Baker's Breakfast Cookies, and so forth. (Refer to Chapter 8 for a complete list of carbohydrate-containing foods.) The type of carbohydrates that you ingest is important. For example, carb-laden foods such as cakes, pies, cookies, candy are not considered good quality. These are very high in refined sugar and will not get you on your path to optimum fitness. In Chapters 8 and 9 I have provided numerous examples of carb-containing foods that are good quality. I give examples that you can eat in restaurants. As I mentioned before, this plan is easy to follow. I want you to become a believer, as my clients have, that good quality carbohydrates are essential in order to reach optimum fitness.

Proteins

Protein is another critical macronutrient. Your muscles are made of proteins. Protein is essential for muscle repair and recovery. When you work out, whether by weight training or cardiovascular exercise, you are tearing your body down. As I learned in my human physiology studies, exercise creates microscopic tears in your muscles. In order to repair this damage, you must ingest protein.

Good sources include: lean meats, fish, egg whites, egg substitutes, protein powders (Champion Nutrition Whey Protein, Champion Nutrition ULTRAMET lite...refer to Chapter 10), soy protein meatless products, skim milk, soy milk, low-fat cottage cheese, low-fat cheese, and so on. (Refer to Chapter 8 for a complete list of protein-containing foods.)

Fats

Fat is a word that does not seem to fit into a nutrition and fitness program. Believe it or not, dietary fats are one of your most critical macronutrients. Most of the cells in our body are made of fats; therefore, incorporating proper fats into our nutrition can help nourish our skin, hair, and nails.

Saturated fats, such as those coming from sweets, chocolates, fried foods, and fast foods, are not the fats I am speaking of; they make the body produce more cholesterol, which may raise blood cholesterol levels. Excess saturated fat is related to an increased risk of cardiovascular disease. Unsaturated fats are the "good" fats you need to incorporate into your diet. These fats come from certain oils, nuts, peanut butter, Power PB (refer to Chapter10), and omega-3 fatty acids (found in certain types of fish such as salmon).

It is critical to eat good dietary fats (unsaturated) in order to burn our stored body fat. Eating unsaturated fats is not only healthy, but they will also satisfy our hunger mechanism. It is this satiation that will greatly reduce one's cravings for the "not so good" foods.

The key to changing your lifestyle is to keep the beneficial balance of carbohydrates, proteins, and fats that I will demonstrate to you in Chapter 8. The goal of proper nutrition is to stabilize your blood sugar throughout the day. If you were to eat only a plate of pasta and then test your blood sugar, you would notice a rapid and significant rise in your blood sugar. Following this rise in blood sugar will be a rapid drop in your blood sugar. Your energy levels will follow this same path with this rise and fall in blood sugar. As your blood sugar rises, so will your energy levels. As your blood sugar falls, you will become tired and lethargic.

Have you ever experienced an "afternoon lull" in the middle of your workday? If so, you most likely experienced a significant drop in your blood sugar.

Imagine if you could prevent these drops in your blood sugar throughout the day. It would only make sense that your energy levels would remain high, right? This is exactly right. If you are like most people, you would like to have more energy throughout your day. I have put my biochemistry and physiology knowledge to work for you. This is exactly what my nutrition is designed to do. Through proper nutrition, you will teach your body to stabilize your blood sugar, thereby creating a much higher and stable energy level throughout the day. In order to achieve optimum fitness and to become forever fit, increasing your energy levels is critical. As previously mentioned, increased energy is one of the wonderful dynamics you will experience with your lifestyle change. If you are prepared for increased energy levels, read on!

2
Nutrition

Increasing Your Metabolism

You hear a lot of talk about metabolism. Those individuals always trying to lose weight are complaining that they have a "slow" metabolism. These are the same individuals who feel that all fit people are fit because they are lucky due to their "fast" metabolism. Refer back to Chapter 2, where I talked about "stinkin' thinkin'. These last two statements refer back to this. If this is your thinking, let's change it right now. If you feel your metabolism is slow, it is most likely due to poor nutritional or exercise habits. Throughout this book, I have had you change your thinking on a number of issues such as having a positive attitude regarding your goal-dreams and your thinking regarding carbohydrates. Now it is time to change your thinking regarding your metabolism.

Each and every one of us has a Basal Metabolic Rate (BMR). This refers to the amount of calories we can burn at rest without any physical activity. The leaner (lower percentage of body fat) someone is, the higher his or her BMR, therefore more calories will be burned at rest. The reason some people have a "slow" metabolism (aside from certain glandular deficiencies) is due to their poor nutritional habits. The opposite is true as well. Those individuals with a "fast" metabolism have created this through a good quality nutrition and fitness regimen.

Let's take a look at a very common scenario that I have seen with the majority of clients I have coached. As I mentioned before, one of the biggest problems I see is that those looking to lose weight do not eat enough. Take that person who skips breakfast each morning. Let's say this individual eats dinner at 7:00 PM each night and gets up at 6:00 AM each morning and goes off to work without eating breakfast. Their first meal may not come until noon. Remember, this person last ate at 7:00 PM the night before. This is a seventeen-hour fast that this individual just experienced. Seventeen hours and no food! (Granted, this person was sleeping for six to eight hours; therefore, nine to eleven waking hours transpired without food.) Some of you may be thinking a fast like this is good for losing weight. By not eating, weight loss is likely to occur, right? Wrong. If this situation describes you, do not worry. It can be fixed. Even if you are afraid of eating breakfast because you are not hungry, you can change your thinking. If you are not hungry upon awakening, there is an explanation for this.

Physiologically, our body is very smart. When we "starve'" our bodies, as in the abovementioned fast, our body perceives this as a dangerous situation. Our body senses this lack of food intake and goes into "starvation mode." So, what do you think is happening to your metabolism at this time? If you said slowing down, you are correct. The body will automatically slow your metabolism to counteract this "starvation" you are putting it through. The body does not want to burn more calories because it feels threatened by not being fed.

Think of your metabolism, or calorie burning, on a scale of 0–10, where 0 equals no calorie burning, and 10 equals highest possible calorie burning. Let's say your metabolism normally burns at a level 5 and almost every day you skip breakfast. Keep in mind how smart your body is. Your body cannot possibly continue to burn at a level 5 because it feels as if it is being "starved." In order to protect you from withering away, your body may slow to a level 3. Now you have just slowed your metabolism due to poor nutritional habits. The real problem comes in when this occurs not just for days, but for months and years.

There is a cumulative effect in terms of your metabolism. The longer you continue to "starve" your body, the slower your metabolism. Your body and its metabolism will not work for you unless you work for your body. Eating, the proper food of course, is viewed by the body as work. The body has been fed; therefore it has work to do. It wants to digest the food and the metabolism begins to turn on. If you work for your body and treat it right, it will work for you.

Remember the individual I mentioned who tries to lose weight by skipping breakfast? They usually follow the same pattern throughout the day: Skip breakfast; eat a substantial lunch and a *very* large dinner that may continue late into the night. This is a true recipe for disaster. Hunger will strike and strike big late in the day due to the early starvation mode. Refer back to Chapter 6, where I talked about stabilizing your blood sugar. When you skip breakfast your blood sugar will drop. You will then get a moderate rise and a subsequent fall in blood sugar following your moderate lunch. Then, come dinnertime, when you want to eat everything in front of you, your blood sugar skyrockets once again. So, to compound the problem, not only are you "starving" your body, but you are also placing your body through huge blood sugar swings throughout the day. I think you will now start to put the pieces of the puzzle together. If you "starve" your body and your blood sugar is out of control, you now realize why your fitness results have been significantly slowed. I previously mentioned that patience is going to be a big key to success. I cannot stress this enough. If you have slowed your metabolism for some time due to the above situation, it will take time to undo this process and get your metabolism back on track. If you believe it, you can achieve it! This is a life plan for you to achieve optimum fitness.

Think of it like this…when you eat, this alerts your body that it must go to work. It is time for your body to start burning calories. Eating turns on the body's light switch. It triggers your body's alarm clock. Your body now has work (digestion) to do. This is what keeps your body's metabolism in high gear. As previously mentioned, just the opposite occurs when we starve ourselves…the body's alarm never gets turned on. Now the body says, "Hey, you did not feed me; therefore, I am not going to work for you." This work is your metabolism. Now, you have just slowed your own metabolism by starving yourself. Put good, clean calories in your system, and your body will reward you by revving up its metabolism and start working for you.

As previously mentioned, both scenarios have cumulative effects. The process of "starving" your body by not feeding it continues to slow your metabolism. As you continue this vicious cycle (starve, slow metabolism, starve, slow metabolism), your body weight continues to increase and your energy levels drop. This usually occurs despite an increase in one's exercise program.

What adds fuel to the fire in the above scenario and continues to slow your metabolism is exercise. No, this does not give you the right to say, "See, I knew exercise was overrated." Let me explain…since your metabolism is already slowed due to insufficient calories, the body will burn fewer calories during exercise. In summary, you are now eating less, working out more, and *not* losing weight. Does this sound familiar? Congratulations, you have just created an extremely inefficient fat burning system within your own body. No worries…I will help you restore that broken-down furnace into an efficient, fat-burning machine.

Let's now examine the flip side of this situation. The individual that does not put his or her body into a caloric deficit will experience just the opposite. Remember, either situation has cumulative effects. The efficient furnace has been built and this person has created a fat burning machine inside. Not only does the "well-fed" individual burn calories during exercise, but twenty-four hours per day. Yes, you heard me right, twenty-four hours per day, even while sleeping. The "well-fed" person will notice a greater body weight loss and body fat loss as opposed to the "starved" person. Why? The reason is a higher metabolism allows a person, even at rest, to burn more calories. An increased metabolism, increased caloric burn translates into one thing…the loss of body weight and body fat.

Nutritional balance is the key. As you will read in Chapter 8, moderation will bring about success. The body needs to be fed small nutritious meals throughout the day. This will create a more stable blood sugar, thereby, minimizing intense food cravings. When we let our body go for hours on end without food, our blood sugar drops drastically. This is when we start to crave foods that are not nutritious. Eating, following a long "starvation" period causes our blood sugar to spike. Following this pattern all day long causes a constant fluctuation in our blood sugar. We can avoid this by simply eating small meals and snacks throughout the day.

I will feel as if I have done my job if I can get you to change your thinking regarding food and eating. Many overweight people who have battled their weight their whole life view food as their enemy. At anytime in their life, if they ate food, they seemed to gain weight. This is the most common situation I have dealt with in my thirteen years of nutrition and fitness coaching. So, please do not feel alone if this is your story. This is more common than not.

You want to lose weight and body fat and your thinking in the past has been crash diets, fad diets, calorie restriction diets, "fat burning" pills, and so on. None of these options include adding food, but just the opposite. You have been told in the past that you must cut out foods to lose weight. Now you are reading that in order for you achieve your goal-dreams and to become forever fit you need to eat, not starve yourself.

As I mentioned earlier, change is not easy. I want you to change your thinking and stop being afraid of eating. Food is not your enemy; rather it is your friend. Review the examples above…starvation will slow your metabolism while eating the proper foods will increase your metabolism, causing a loss of body weight and body fat. The key will be your food choices and your frequency of meals and snacks (refer to Chapter 8). By combining carbohydrates, proteins, and fats for each meal and snack, you will stabilize your blood sugar. This stabilization will prevent your energy swings throughout the day, keeping your energy high and stable. Also, your frequency of eating is critical. If you tend to skip breakfast, you must change your thinking. You will learn to eat 4–6 meals and snacks per day that will contribute to a stable blood sugar, high energy levels, and a high metabolism.

If you are like most individuals, your daily nutrition revolves around a large dinner. As previously mentioned, this is common due to a light to nonexistent breakfast and lunch. This creates an extreme hunger come dinnertime. Once you change your lifestyle, improve your food choices, and improve your frequency of eating, your thinking of dinner will drastically change. Of course, you will still eat dinner; it just will not be your "showcase" meal. Once again, I realize change is not easy. You have your goal-dreams written down and you want to achieve optimum fitness. It is going to be your burning desire to reach your goal-dreams that will make this change easier than expected.

With that said, what is the bottom line? I do not want you to be afraid of carbohydrates, nor do I want you to have a fear of eating. You must eat to lose weight and body fat. If this does not excite you, you should probably put this book down right now. Yes, you can eat well and lose weight. You do *not* need to starve yourself to achieve your goal-dreams and optimum fitness.

Nutrition Program and Guidelines

Of the three phases in this program, (nutrition, weight training, cardiovascular exercise), proper nutrition is the key. With that being said, this will be your *only* focus for the first week of the program. Therefore, if you are already involved in a training program or if you are not presently exercising, I do not want you to start your *new* fitness program until you have completed your first week of *Forever Fit* nutrition. You can continue your present workout program during this first week. I believe in crawling before walking. Let's get your nutrition under way, and then we will start your new fitness program.

I have made the nutrition quite simple. I have your foods broken down into carbohydrates, proteins, fats, and vegetables. Ideally, you want to eat 4–6 meals and snacks each day. For each meal or snack, you will choose one food in each category (carbohydrate, protein, and fat: to be discussed later in the chapter).

Let's review why you always want to eat a combination of carbohydrates, protein, and fat (for additional information, please refer back to Chapter 7):

1. This will keep your blood sugar stable throughout the day, thereby reducing nonnutritious food cravings.

2. This will keep you satiated until it is time for your next meal or snack.

3. This will allow you to increase your metabolism, thereby burning more calories throughout the day (keep in mind, eating burns calories!).

4. Your mental and physical energy will be at an all-time high by eliminating extreme blood sugar fluctuations.

Consider vegetables as an added bonus to your nutrition program. Vegetables will not add much to your overall carbohydrate, protein, and fat totals. They are simply good for you and they promote good health. Adding one serving of vegetables 2–4 times per day will promote good health. If vegetables such as spinach, broccoli, cauliflower, carrots are not accessible, 8 oz. of vegetable or tomato juice is a great alternative (use a low-sodium vegetable juice if sodium intake is a concern to you). One way I teach my clients to get good quality vegetables is in their salads. Try to replace all of your iceberg lettuce with spinach. Spinach contains a high amount of antioxidants. This is important as an anti-carcinogenic (anti-cancer) agent and numerous ophthalmologic studies show that spinach is very good for promoting good ocular (eye) health. As a doctor of optometry, I want to keep your eyes as healthy as possible.

Consult your physician prior to starting your new nutrition program. If you are on diabetic or high blood pressure medications, you may be able to reduce or even eliminate these medications over time. Specific suggestions marked with an asterisk are covered more thoroughly in Chapter 10.

Carbohydrates:

*   1 serving of oatmeal (made with water, soy milk, or skim milk)

*   1–2 slices of bread (preferably wheat…1 slice if approximately 25 g carbohydrates, 2 slices if approximately 13 g carbohydrates)

*   1–2 pieces of fruit

- 1 serving of low-fat soup (non-cream based)
- 1 serving of low-fat yogurt (maximum of 20–25 grams of carbohydrates)
- 1 low-fat or whole wheat frozen waffle
- 1/2–1 Baker's Breakfast Cookie*
- 1/2–1 serving rice (preferably whole grain)
- 1/2–1 serving of pasta
- 1/2 baked or sweet potato
- 1 serving of Champion Nutrition METABOLOL II (MET-2)*

Protein:
- 4–8 oz. chicken
- 4–8 oz. lean red meat
- 4–8 oz. lean pork
- 4–8 oz. fish
- 1/2 can of tuna (in water)
- 2–4 egg whites or egg substitutes
- 1–1 1/2 soy protein/vegetable burger (be sure that in one serving the protein is higher than the carbohydrates, if not this will *not* serve as a protein source)
- 2–3 slices of 2% cheese
- 1 serving low-fat cottage cheese
- 1 serving of Champion Nutrition Pure Whey protein powder (blended with water, skim milk, or soy milk)
- 1 serving of Champion Nutrition ULTRMET lite*
- 1 serving of Champion Nutrition MET-2*

Fats:
- 2 tsp (teaspoon) Power PB or 2 tsp peanut butter

- 1/2 serving nuts (not candy coated or honey roasted)
- 1/2 serving oil (extra-virgin olive oil, safflower, flax seed oil, etc.)
- Low-fat or lite salad dressings (avoid milk-based dressings)
- 1 serving of Champion Nutrition MET-2*

Vegetables:
- 1 serving carrots, peas, broccoli, cauliflower, spinach, or something similar.
- 1 serving vegetable or tomato juice

Meal replacements and pre- and postworkout supplements:
- 1 serving of Champion Nutrition ULTRMET lite*
- 1 serving of Champion Nutrition MET-2*
- 1/2–1 Baker's Breakfast Cookie

Add-ons:
- Ketchup
- Mustard
- Salt free seasoning blends
- Low-fat butter substitutes (powders, sprays, etc.)
- Low-fat cheese substitutes (powders)
- Fat-free cream (plain or flavored), skim milk, 2% milk (for coffee, etc.)

Nutrition Guidelines

- Eat 4–6 meals and snacks per day. Most days, dinner will be your last meal. Depending on how early you eat dinner or how hungry you are, you can add a snack following dinner. Be sure you are not eating just to eat. Listen to your body and learn your body's signals. If you are truly hungry following dinner, you want to eat…just be sure it is not just out of boredom.

- For each meal and snack per day, choose *one* food in each category (carbohydrate, protein, fat).

- Drink a minimum of 64 oz. of water per day…Penta water* (this is in addition to water consumed during exercise).

- Utilize liquid supplements such as MET-2 and ULTRAMET lite as snacks (this will deliver good quality carbohydrates and protein and fat, thereby diminishing food cravings).

- The program is designed for you to get hungry every few hours. Use the "grazing" philosophy…you will be eating small meals and snacks all throughout the day.

- Hunger is *not* a bad sign. This actually means the body is responding properly to your new lifestyle of small and frequent meals all throughout the day. Hunger is a sign that your metabolism has been jump-started and calories and body fat are being burned up.

- Keep in mind that you want to eat just enough to satiate (this is the feeling following a meal that your hunger has been satisfied) yourself, but not to overfill yourself. After each meal or snack, you should simply feel satiated, *not* overstuffed.

Forever Fit Meal Plan

___/___/___ a.m. weight=___ p.m. weight=___ body fat___%

	<u>Carbohydrate</u>	<u>Protein</u>	<u>Fat</u>
B Plan			
B Actual			
S1 Plan			
S1 Actual			
L Plan			
L Actual			

S2 Plan
S2 Actual

D Plan
D Actual

S3 Plan
S3 Actual

Notes:

B= Breakfast
L= Lunch
D= Dinner
S= Snack

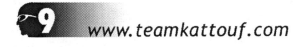

Forever Fit Sample Meals and Snacks

Note: Try to incorporate approximately two fruits and two servings of vegetables (or 8 oz. vegetable or tomato juice) each day. A salad with vegetables is considered one serving of vegetables.

Note: Any carbohydrate listed can be substituted with 1–2 pieces of fruit (i.e., apple, orange, pear, plum, banana, etc.)

Note: 2 tsp peanut butter can be substituted for Power PB

Menu samples:
Breakfast:

1 serving oatmeal or cereal
Protein drink (approx 20 g)
2 tsp Power PB

1 serving oatmeal or cereal
1 serving low-fat cottage cheese
2 tsp Power PB

1 serving oatmeal or cereal
2–4 egg substitutes or egg whites
2 tsp Power PB

1–2 slices wheat bread
1 serving low-fat cottage cheese
2 tsp Power PB

1–2 slices wheat bread
2–4 egg substitutes or egg whites
2 tsp Power PB

1–2 slices wheat bread
Protein drink
2 tsp Power PB

1/2 Baker's Breakfast Cookie
Protein drink
2 tsp Power PB

1/2 Baker's Breakfast Cookie
1 serving low-fat cottage cheese
2 tsp Power PB

1/2 Baker's Breakfast Cookie
2–4 egg substitutes or egg whites
2 tsp Power PB

1–2 fruit
1 serving cottage cheese or 2–4 egg substitutes or egg whites or 1 protein drink
2 tsp Power PB

Lunch:

1 bowl soup (non-cream based)
Grilled chicken or tuna salad
Low-fat dressing or oil and vinegar

2 slices wheat bread
Grilled chicken
Salad with low-fat dressing or oil and vinegar

2 slices wheat bread
1/2 can tuna
Salad with low-fat dressing or oil and vinegar

1–2 slices of bread or rolls
Grilled chicken or tuna salad
Low-fat dressing or oil and vinegar

2 slices wheat bread
1–1.5 soy protein burger
Salad with low-fat dressing or oil and vinegar

1 yogurt
1 serving cottage cheese
2 tsp Power PB

6" sub with lunchmeat or chicken
Add vegetables
Cheese or oil will serve as fat

1/2 burrito with chicken or steak and beans
Cheese will serve as fat
If you add rice, omit the tortilla

1/2 sandwich with lunchmeat
1/2 salad with chicken
Cheese will serve as fat

1–2 fruit
1 serving low-fat cottage cheese
2 tsp Power PB

Dinner:

1 serving rice
Chicken or fish or meat
1 serving vegetables
Salad w/non- or low-fat dressing

1/2 potato (baked or sweet)
Chicken/fish/meat
1 serving vegetables
Salad with non- or low-fat dressing

1 serving pasta
Chicken/fish/meat
1 serving vegetables
Salad w/non-low-fat dressing

1 serving rice
1–2 soy protein burgers
1 serving vegetables
Salad with low-fat dressing or oil and vinegar

1/2 potatoes
1–2 soy protein burgers
1 serving vegetables
Salad with low-fat dressing or oil and vinegar

1 bowl soup
Chicken/fish/meat
Salad w/non-low-fat dressing
1 serving vegetables

1 serving pasta
1–2 soy protein burgers
1 serving vegetables
Salad w/non-low-fat dressing

Snacks:

1 fruit
Protein drink
2 tsp Power PB

1 yogurt
1 serving cottage cheese
2 tsp Power PB

1/2 Baker's Breakfast Cookie
Protein drink
2 tsp Power PB

1 fruit
1 serving low-fat cottage cheese
2 tsp Power PB

1 fruit
1 serving ULTRAMET lite
2 tsp Power PB

1/2 Baker's Breakfast Cookie
1 serving ULTRAMET lite
2 tsp Power PB

1 Baker's Breakfast Cookie
or 1 serving MET-2

Everyone has a unique schedule. Some individuals like to work out first thing in the morning, others at lunchtime, while others can only find time after work. In order to keep this nutrition program as easy to follow as possible, I will cover all three scenarios. In each situation you may be faced with challenges. I want to take the thinking out of this so you can simply follow the nutrition as prescribed and enjoy the results.

If you choose to work out first thing in the morning:

6:00 AM Pre-workout:

1 serving of Champion Nutrition MET-2

7:30 AM Breakfast:

1 serving oatmeal
1 serving Champion Nutrition Whey protein
2 tsp Power PB

10:00 AM Snack:

1 Baker's Breakfast Cookie

12:00 PM Lunch:

Grilled chicken sandwich
Salad with low-fat dressing or oil and vinegar
8 oz vegetable juice

2:00 PM:

1 Go Fast light

3:00 PM Snack:

1 fruit
1 serving cottage cheese
2 tsp Power PB

6:00 PM Dinner:

1 serving rice
Chicken/fish/meat

Salad with low-fat dressing or oil and vinegar
8 oz vegetable juice

8:30 PM Snack (Optional):

1 fruit
1 serving Champion Nutrition Whey protein
2 tsp Power PB

If you choose to work out at lunchtime:

7:00 AM Breakfast:

1–2 fruit
1 serving low-fat cottage cheese
2 tsp Power PB

10:00 AM Snack:

1 Baker's Breakfast Cookie

11:45 PM Pre-workout:

1/2 serving Champion Nutrition MET-2 (Only 1/2 serving because the
Baker's cookie was eaten at 10:00)
1 Go Fast regular

12:00 PM workout:

1:00 PM Lunch:

6" sub with chicken or lunchmeat, vegetables and either oil or cheese
8 oz vegetable juice

3:00 PM Snack:

1 fruit
1 serving Champion Nutrition Whey protein
2 tsp Power PB

6:00 PM Dinner:

1 bowl soup
Chicken/fish/meat

Salad with low-fat dressing or oil
8 oz vegetable juice

8:30 PM Snack (Optional):

1 yogurt
1 serving Champion Nutrition Whey protein
2 tsp Power PB

If you choose to work out after work:

7:00 AM Breakfast:

1–2 slices wheat bread
1 serving low-fat cottage cheese
2 tsp Power PB

10:00 AM Snack:

1 Baker's Breakfast Cookie

12:00 PM Lunch:

1/2 sandwich with chicken or lunchmeat
1/2 salad with chicken and cheese w/nonfat dressing
8 oz vegetable juice

3:00 PM Snack:

1 fruit
1 serving Champion Nutrition ULTRAMET lite
2 tsp Power PB

5:30 PM Pre-workout:

1 serving Champion Nutrition MET-2
1 Go Fast regular or light

7:30 PM Dinner:

1/2 potato
Chicken/fish/meat

Salad with low-fat dressing
1 serving vegetables

9:00 PM Snack (Optional):

1 fruit
1 serving Champion Nutrition Whey protein
2 tsp Power PB

Due to busy schedules and sheer convenience, many of you will choose to eat at restaurants. As throughout this entire book my goal is to simplify the *Forever Fit* nutrition for you, making it easy to follow. I want you to be able to "live" and follow my program simultaneously. Keep in mind, *Forever Fit* is a life plan, not a diet; therefore, you need to be able to continue this lifestyle even after you meet and exceed your goals. Let's take a look at some sample meals that you can order at restaurants while meeting your carbohydrate, protein, and fat needs. I will break this down for you into breakfasts, lunches, and dinners at different restaurant types. Enjoy eating out without the guilt!

Breakfast eateries:

1 order wheat toast (no butter)
2–4 egg substitutes
2 tsp Power PB

1 order wheat toast
Egg substitute omelet with cheese and vegetables (mushrooms, tomatoes, peppers, etc.)
Cheese will serve as your fat

1 order wheat toast (no butter)
2–4 eggs
Eggs will serve as your protein and fat

1 order wheat toast (no butter)
Vegetable omelet
Eggs will serve as your protein and fat

1 pancake
2–4 egg substitutes
Pancake will serve as your carbohydrate and fat

1 order oatmeal
Egg substitute vegetable omelet with cheese
Cheese will serve as your fat

Lunch and dinner:
Sandwich eateries:

6" wheat sub with lunchmeat, cheese, and vegetables
You can substitute oil for cheese as your fat

6" wheat sub with chicken, cheese, and vegetables
You can substitute oil for cheese as your fat

Sandwich wrap with chicken, vegetables, and cheese
You can substitute oil for cheese

1/2 burrito with chicken or steak and beans and vegetables
If you choose to add rice, omit the tortilla

1/2 sandwich with chicken or lunchmeat
1/2 salad with chicken, cheese, and non- or low-fat dressing

1/2 sandwich with chicken or lunchmeat and cheese
Soup (non-cream based)

Steak eateries:

1 roll or piece of bread
Grilled chicken or steak salad
Low-fat or lite dressing

1 bowl soup
Grilled chicken or steak salad
Low-fat or lite dressing

1 serving rice
Grilled chicken and steamed vegetables
Salad with low-fat or lite dressing

1 serving rice
Fish (not fried) and steamed vegetables
Salad with low-fat or lite dressing

1/2 potato
4–10 oz. steak and steamed vegetables
Salad with nonfat, low-fat, lite dressing

1 serving rice
4–10 oz. steak and steamed vegetables
Salad with nonfat, low-fat, or lite dressing

Italian eateries:

The key to eating at Italian eateries is to pick your protein as your primary meal and your carbohydrate secondary. The reason behind this is to keep your carbohydrates and proteins from being out of balance. When you order a pasta and chicken dish, you get an abundance of pasta and very little chicken. This becomes a "carbohydrate heavy" meal. A better choice is to order a chicken dish and get a side of pasta. This keeps the carbohydrates and proteins in balance.

Side of pasta with tomato or marinara sauce
Grilled chicken breast or chicken marsala
Salad with low-fat or lite dressing

1 bowl soup
Grilled chicken breast or chicken marsala with steamed vegetables
Salad with low-fat or lite dressing

1–2 slices *thin* crust pizza with chicken and vegetables
Salad with nonfat or lite dressing
Cheese on the pizza will serve as your fat
The thin crust will allow you to keep your carbohydrates and protein in balance

1 slice thin crust cheese pizza
Salad with chicken and low-fat or lite dressing
Cheese on pizza will serve as your fat

1–2 breadsticks without butter (ask your server to have them made without butter)
Grilled chicken breast or chicken marsala with steamed vegetables
Salad with low-fat or lite dressing

1–2 breadsticks without butter (ask your server to have them made with-out butter…he or she will be more than happy to do this for you)
Grilled chicken breast salad with cheese and low-fat or lite dressing
Cheese will serve as your fat

The following is one of my signature meals at my favorite local Italian eatery:
Side of pasta with grilled chicken, spinach, mushrooms, and tomatoes all tossed in a chicken broth
Salad with low-fat or lite dressing

Yes, ask your server and they will mix this in chicken broth. You may get a strange look, but when the meal arrives you will love the taste!

10 www.teamkattouf.com

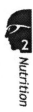

Nutritional Secret Weapons

Throughout my life, I have tried a lot of nutrition products. I look at a number of factors when it comes to nutrition product. Taste is very important. If something tastes good you will obviously be much more inclined to eat it. Ease of use is important as well. I want a product I can not only have at home and work, but also travel with. If you find something that is nutritious and you can eat it on a daily basis, this will allow you to stay on track nutritionally even when you travel. Another important factor is making sure the product contributes to the goals at hand: increased energy, weight loss, and body fat loss, which all lead to improved self-esteem. In this chapter you will read about nine fabulous nutrition products that will assist you in achieving optimum fitness. For more information, please visit www.teamkattouf.com. Note: Several of the products mentioned in this section sponsor my athletic competition, and for this I owe them a debt of gratitude. But my endorsement of their products is not just based on my experience using them, but also the experiences of my clients. If they can help everyday people reach optimum fitness, I'm sure they can help you!

Power PB: Once you taste Power PB, you won't ever go back to ordinary peanut butter! Power PB is made for athletes of any sport, at any level. Its highly effective peanut-based protein nutrient supplement replenishes muscle and calories burned after your workout. Power PB is a safe and effective source of dietary fat, and provides you with high-quality unsaturated fat. It contains flaxseed, flaxseed oil, omega-3 and omega-6 fatty acids, and egg whites. Many of my clients have incorporated Power PB into their fitness 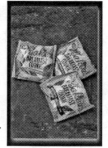 regimens because of its smooth taste and protein-rich ingredients. I use Power PB all throughout the day as my source of fat. It is great to travel with when I go to a race. I even take some with me if I go to a restaurant. This stuff rocks…it's what peanut butter should be. To order Power PB, turn to Appendix A.

Baker's Breakfast Cookie: Baker's got it right! Hands down, this is the finest tasting energy cookie available. Baker's Breakfast Cookies are all natural and great tasting. These things sell themselves. At the fitness center where I teach spinning, Q-Club Fitness in Warren, Ohio, these cookies are flying off the shelf. This little cookie has become very popular with many of my clients, and I'm not surprised (I have a drawer in my office filled with them!). They are great between breakfast and lunch as well as between lunch and dinner. You can travel with them. Be sure to keep some at work as well as in your car. Baker's Breakfast Cookies make planning your daily nutrition easy. Vegan Peanut Butter Chocolate Chunk is my favorite. I choose to store mine in the refrigerator, then warm it up for 18–20 seconds in the microwave. If you store them at room temperature, 7–8 seconds in the microwave will do the trick. If you have a sweet tooth, these babies are the answer.

Here is a quick story about this product. A friend of mine at Q-Club Fitness (let's refer to him as Bill Jones) followed my lead and incorporated Baker's Breakfast Cookies into his daily nutrition. Prior to eating the cookies, Bill found himself eating less, skipping breakfast, working out more, and gaining weight. Bill then tried Baker's Breakfast Cookie. The only thing Bill changed in his daily nutrition was he stopped skipping breakfast. Instead, he ate a cookie every morning. Bill continued his present workout routine that consisted of 4–6 days per week of weight training and cardiovascular exercise. Bill said that Baker's cookies were the only change he had made to his nutrition. The result...Bill lost an amazing 25 lbs. His coworkers got word of this and to this day refer to it as the "Jones' cookie diet." (Refer to Chapter 7 in regards to the importance of breakfast). To order Baker's Breakfast Cookies, turn to appendix A.

Go Fast: With the nationwide craze of energy drinks, one is heads and shoulders above the rest...Go Fast Energy Drink. With better flavor, more active ingredients, lower sodium and sugars, and no preservatives, this is the premium energy drink on the market. Lightly carbonated, refreshing, and flavored with Australian honey instead of high fructose corn syrup, Go Fast has a great taste without a medicinal flavor or aftertaste. Its active ingredients include taurine, caffeine, ginseng, guarana, ginkgo biloba, vitamin B6, vitamin 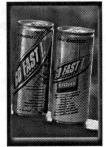 B12, vitamin B3 (niacin), vitamin B8 (pantothenic acid), inositol, and milk thistle herb. You now have two Go Fast options, Go Fast regular and Go Fast light. My clients truly enjoy this product. It is the number one energy drink requested at Q-Club Fitness. I use Go Fast regular prior to working out and racing. Go Fast light is good to use midday as it has lower sugar content. Keep in mind, Go Fast is not used in place of any carbohydrate source in your nutrition program; it is simply used in addition to your daily nutrition. To order Go Fast, turn to Appendix A.

Champion Nutrition MET-2: This is a great tasting, balanced meal supplement designed to assist in increasing your metabolism. MET-2 is ideal for people of all ages. Whether you have digestive disorders, which can cause you to experience an upset stomach or nausea, or you simply need a balanced meal on the go, MET-2 is for you. You can use it to start your day or as a snack. It contains an ideal balance of carbohydrates, proteins, and fats. MET-2 is a calori- 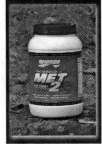 cally efficient food that can help you lose weight without losing muscle mass. I use MET-2 during the day at my office and in the morning prior to working out. My clients have found this to be very valuable for their nutrition and fitness program. My favorite flavor is orange smoothie. Just mix the MET-2 powder with water, shake it in a bottle, and you have a complete meal. To order MET-2, turn to Appendix A.

Champion Nutrition Pure Whey Protein: We all have busy lives, and it is often difficult to have protein sources readily available. Pure Whey is your answer. Use this as your protein source for any meal or snack. As with MET-2, just mix with water and enjoy. Pure Whey can help your body burn fat. I use this all throughout the day as my protein source. I keep it at work and home. My clients have found that Pure Whey makes following the nutrition program even easier. They are not guessing as to what they should use for a 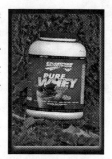 protein source. Discover your favorite flavor and enjoy. I like to mix 1/2 scoop Banana Scream with 1/2 scoop Cocoa-Mochaccino...the taste rocks! To order Whey Protein, turn to Appendix A.

Champion Nutrition ULTRAMET lite: Another great source of protein to use at home, work, or on the go. Containing a combination of casein and whey protein, as well as around 17 g of carbohydrates, ULTRAMET lite will help boost your metabolism. Since ULTRAMET lite has some carbohydrates, you simply can add a "light" carbohydrate (such as a piece of fruit, 1/2 Baker's Breakfast Cookie or a Baker's Breakfast Cookie mini), 2 tsp of Power PB, and you have a power-packed meal or snack. I enjoy a chocolate 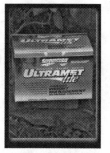 ULTRAMET lite shake, 1/2 a Baker's Breakfast Cookie, and Power PB anytime of the day. This gives me the energy I am seeking. To order ULTRAMET lite, turn to Appendix A.

Penta: No chemicals are ever used to purify Penta water. This is the purest bottled water available (even purer than distilled water). Due to Penta's unique properties, it has a smaller molecular makeup than ordinary water, and it moves through the body quickly for superior hydration. Penta water is the best tasting water and seems to be a very "clean and pure" water. I keep multiple cases at my office and home. I make sure Penta is with me at all times during traveling.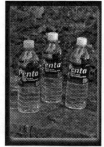

MaxiVision: We all need a good quality multiple vitamin supplement. After extensive research, I found the best product available: MaxiVision Whole Body Formula. It provides you with nutrients to benefit both the ocular (eye) system and the whole body. There has been extensive research on the benefits of lutein, a powerful antioxidant for the eye. Research shows that 6 mg of lutein per day can help prevent macular degeneration (a blinding eye condition), and 10–20 mg of lutein per day can actually stabilize and reverse some 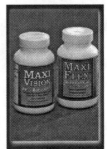 of the changes associated with macular degeneration. MaxiVision Whole Body Formula provides you with 20 mg of lutein per day in a multivitamin format (the highest lutein content of any product). Compare MaxiVision to your present multivitamin and you will see the difference. This is my daily multivitamin. Many patients and clients of mine have realized the benefits of MaxiVision. Please consult with your physician prior to taking any multivitamin. To order MaxiVision, turn to Appendix A.

MaxiFlex: You may have read about glucosamine and chondroitin. These supplements have been touted as a natural anti-inflammatory to help maintain joint function. MaxiFlex goes beyond the other products on the market. Aside from containing glucosamine and chondroitin, it also contains MSM. This supplement has proved very valuable for me on a daily basis. Patients and clients of mine have discovered the wonderful benefits that MaxiFlex provides. Try it for yourself. To order MaxiFlex, turn to Appendix A.

I am sure you will enjoy these products as much as my patients, my clients, my acquaintances, and I have. As previously mentioned, proper nutrition is the key to success. Focus on the nutrition, see the results, and feel the increased energy. These products will help make your goal-dreams reality!

Section III:
Weight Training and
Cardiovascular Exercise

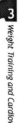

Weight Training Program

There may be some misconceptions in regards to weight training. Many individuals feel that in order to lose weight, cardiovascular exercise needs to be increased significantly. Cardiovascular exercise is clearly important for weight loss and body fat loss, but weight training may produce a greater body fat loss when properly combined in a good quality fitness program like the one you are about to begin.

Weight training will build lean muscle tissue. Muscle is the highest metabolic tissue in our body. This means that the leaner you are, the more calories you will burn. This is how you increase your metabolism...build lean muscle. If weight training is new to you, you may have to change your thinking about weight training. If you are like a lot of people I have coached, your definition

69

of weight training is similar to that of bodybuilding. Women especially seem to shy away at first from weight training. I always hear them say that they do not want to get "big muscles." If this is your thinking, you no longer need to worry. I want you to think of weight training as a significant part of your training program that will bring about optimum fitness. Weight training will build lean muscle and burn body fat. Remember, optimum fitness first requires you to have a body fat percentage within the recommended values. Enjoy your weight training, because the results can be nothing short of amazing!

Your weight training program will be based on three days of weight training per week with a fourth optional day. The program will be broken down into three-week blocks. Week one: straight sets. Week two: supersets. Week three: giant sets. Following this three-week block, you will then return to straight sets and repeat.

- **Straight sets:** One set of one exercise is performed, followed by complete rest prior to starting your next exercise. *For example: seated dumbbell bicep curls: 2 sets; 8 reps. Perform 8 reps of bicep curls, rest, and then perform 8 reps bicep curls. This completes the 2 sets.*

- **Supersets:** Two exercises performed back-to-back without rest. *For example: seated dumbbell bicep curls: 2 supersets; 8 reps, 12 reps. Perform 8 reps bicep curls, immediately lighten the weight, and then perform 12 reps bicep curls, rest. This is one superset.*

- **Giant sets:** Three exercises performed back-to-back-to-back *without rest. For example: seated dumbbell bicep curls: 2 giant sets; 8 reps, 10 reps, 12 reps. Perform 8 reps bicep curls, immediately lighten the weight, perform 10 reps bicep curls, immediately lighten the weight, and perform 12 reps bicep curls, rest. This is one giant set.*

Following each three-week block, the goal is to increase the weight used for each exercise. The number of repetitions prescribed will determine the amount of weight that you use. For example, if eight repetitions are prescribed, the amount of weight you use should be such that repetitions six through eight should be challenging but not impossible. If you cannot complete the repetitions prescribed, the weight you chose is too heavy. On the flip side, if you easily complete the repetitions prescribed and you could have performed five–ten more repetitions, you should choose a heavier weight. It may take you a few attempts to dial in the weight to use for each exercise prescribed. Be patient and shortly you will know exactly what weight to use. Being able to increase the weight lifted is a great sign of increased strength. Increased strength equates to the development of lean muscle tissue. Remember, increasing your lean muscle means increasing your body's ability to burn body fat and calories. This dynamic process will not only cause your body to burn fat and calories during exercise, but all throughout the day. So just imagine, as you successfully progress through your weight training program, you are training your body to burn more calories and fat twenty-four hours per day...even at rest.

Weight-Training Tips

- Consult your physician prior to beginning your weight training program.

- Keep in mind, I recommend that you do not begin your new training program until you get a full week of nutrition under your belt. I do not want to overload you with too much new information in the first week. The nutrition is so crucial in order for you to achieve optimum fitness.

- If you are already exercising, simply continue with your present routine during this first week.

- Your weight training program is based on three days per week. If you choose to complete a fourth day (optional) of weight training, you will repeat the upper body weight training day.

- Be sure to stretch (refer to the stretching photos later in this chapter) before and after working out.

- Following week twelve, go back to week one and repeat the weight training program. At this point, you will be more experienced with the weight training. If time permits, you can add a set if you want to increase the intensity of the workout. Also, at this point, you can substitute exercises (refer to photos) that work the same muscles. For example, seated dumbbell bicep curls for straight bar cable bicep curls, wide grip pull downs for wide grip pull-ups, flat bench dumbbell press for flat bench dumbbell fly.

- Be sure to start with lightweight in order to minimize muscle soreness.

- Refer to photos for proper form on all exercises.

    Week One: Day 1 and 3…Legs:
    Squats: 2 sets; 12 reps
    Leg Press: 2 sets; 12 reps
    Leg Extension: 2 sets; 12 reps
    Leg Curl: 2 sets; 12 reps
    Calf Raises: 2 sets; 12 reps

    Week One: Day 2…Upper Body:
    Bench Press: 2 sets; 10 reps
    Triceps Extensions: 2 sets; 10 reps
    Seated Dumbbell Bicep Curl: 2 sets; 10 reps
    Wide Grip Pull Downs: 2 sets; 10 reps
    Seated Dumbbell Shoulder Press: 2 sets; 10 reps

    Week One: Day 1, 2, 3…Abs:
    Cable Crunches: 1 set; 15 reps
    Cable Oblique Crunches: 1 set; 15 reps

    Week Two: Day 1 and 3…Legs:
    Leg Extension: 2 supersets; 8 reps, 10 reps
    Leg Press: 2 supersets; 8 reps, 10 reps
    Leg Curl: 2 supersets; 8 reps, 10 reps
    Calf Raises: 2 supersets; 8 reps, 10 reps

    Week Two: Day 2…Upper Body
    Flat Bench Dumbbell Press: 2 supersets; 8 reps, 10 reps
    Triceps Extensions: 2 supersets; 8 reps, 10 reps
    Seated Dumbbell Bicep Curl: 2 supersets; 8 reps, 10 reps
    Wide Grip Pull Downs: 2 supersets; 8 reps, 10 reps
    Seated Dumbbell Shoulder Press: 2 supersets; 8 reps, 10 reps

    Week Two: Day 1, 2, 3…Abs:
    Cable Crunches: 1 set; 25 reps
    Cable Oblique Crunches: 1 set; 25 reps

    Week Three: Day 1 and 3…Legs:
    Leg Extension: 2 giant sets; 8 reps, 10 reps, 12 reps
    Leg Press: 2 giant sets; 8 reps, 10 reps, 12 reps

Leg Curl: 2 giant sets; 8 reps, 10 reps, 12 reps
Calf Raises: 2 giant sets; 8 reps, 10 reps, 12 reps

Week Three: Day 2…Upper Body:
Flat Bench Dumbbell Press: 2 giant sets; 8 reps, 10 reps, 12 reps
Triceps Extensions: 2 giant sets; 8 reps, 10 reps, 12 reps
Seated Bicep Dumbbell Curl: 2 giant sets; 8 reps, 10 reps, 12 reps
Wide Grip Pull Downs: 2 giant sets; 8 reps, 10 reps, 12 reps
Seated Dumbbell Shoulder Press: 2 giant sets; 8 reps, 10 reps, 12 reps

Week Three: Day 1, 2, 3…Abs:
Cable Crunches: 1 set; 25 reps
Cable Oblique Crunches: 1 set; 25 reps

Week Four: Day 1 and 3…Legs:
Squats: 3 sets; 10 reps
Leg Extension: 3 sets; 15 reps
Leg Curl: 3 sets; 15 reps
Calf Raises: 3 sets; 15 reps

Week Four: Day 2…Upper Body:
Bench Press: 3 sets; 8 reps
Seated Dumbbell Bicep Curl: 3 sets; 8 reps
Seated Alternating Dumbbell Press: 3 sets; 8 reps
Triceps Extensions: 3 sets; 8 reps
Wide Grip Pull Downs: 3 sets; 8 reps

Week Four: Day 1, 2, 3…Abs:
Cable Crunches: 2 sets; 15 reps
Cable Oblique Crunches: 2 sets; 15 reps

Week Five: Day 1 and 3…Legs:
Leg Press: 2 supersets; 10 reps, 12 reps
Leg Curl: 2 supersets; 10 reps, 12 reps
Leg Extension: 2 supersets; 10 reps, 12 reps
Calf Raises: 2 supersets; 10 reps, 12 reps

Week Five: Day 2…Upper Body:
Flat Bench Dumbbell Press: 2 supersets; 10 reps, 12 reps
Wide Grip Pull Downs: 2 supersets; 10 reps, 12 reps
Triceps Extensions: 2 supersets; 10 reps, 12 reps

Seated Dumbbell Shoulder Press: 2 supersets; 10 reps, 12 reps
Seated Dumbbell Bicep Curl: 2 supersets; 10 reps, 12 reps

Week Five: Day 1, 2, 3…Abs:
Cable Crunches: 2 sets; 20 reps
Cable Oblique Crunches: 2 sets; 20 reps

Week Six: Day 1 and 3…Legs:
Leg Press: 2 giant sets; 10 reps, 12 reps, 15 reps
Leg Extension: 2 giant sets; 10 reps, 12 reps, 15 reps
Leg Curl: 2 giant sets; 10 reps, 12 reps, 15 reps
Calf Raises: 2 giant sets; 10 reps, 12 reps, 15 reps

Week Six: Day 2…Upper Body:
Flat Bench Dumbbell Press: 2 giant sets; 10 reps, 12 reps, 15 reps
Seated Dumbbell Bicep Curl: 2 giant sets; 10 reps, 12 reps, 15 reps
Triceps Extensions: 2 giant sets; 10 reps, 12 reps, 15 reps
Seated Dumbbell Shoulder Press: 2 giant sets; 10 reps, 12 reps, 15 reps
Wide Grip Pull Downs: 2 giant sets; 10 reps, 12 reps, 15 reps

Week Six: Day 1, 2, 3…Abs:
Cable Crunches: 2 sets; 20 reps
Cable Oblique Crunches: 2 sets; 20 reps

Week Seven: Day 1 and 3…Legs:
Squats: 2 sets; 15 reps
Leg Press: 2 sets; 15 reps
Leg Extension: 2 sets; 15 reps
Leg Curl: 2 sets; 15 reps
Calf Raises: 2 sets; 15 reps

Week Seven: Day 2…Upper Body:
Bench Press: 2 sets; 12 reps
Wide Grip Pull Downs: 2 sets; 12 reps
Seated Dumbbell Bicep Curl: 2 sets; 12 reps
Seated Dumbbell Shoulder Press: 2 sets; 12 reps
Triceps Extensions: 2 sets; 12 reps

Week Seven: Day 1, 2, 3…Abs:
Cable Crunches: 2 sets; 25 reps
Cable Oblique Crunches: 2 sets; 25 reps

Week Eight: Day 1 and 3...Legs:
Leg Extension: 2 supersets; 8 reps, 15 reps
Leg Press: 2 supersets; 8 reps, 15 reps
Leg Curl: 2 supersets; 8 reps, 15 reps
Calf Raises: 2 supersets; 8 reps, 15 reps

Week Eight: Day 2...Upper Body:
Dips: 2 supersets; 8 reps, 15 reps
Seated Dumbbell Bicep Curl: 2 supersets; 8 reps, 15 reps
Triceps Extensions: 2 supersets; 8 reps, 15 reps
Seated Dumbbell Shoulder Press: 2 supersets; 8 reps, 15 reps
Wide Grip Pull Downs: 2 supersets; 8 reps, 15 reps

Week Eight: Day 1, 2, 3...Abs:
Cable Crunches: 3 sets; 20 reps
Cable Oblique Crunches: 3 sets; 20 reps

Week Nine: Day 1 and 3...Legs:
Leg Press: 2 giant sets; 8 reps, 15 reps, 20 reps
Leg Extensions: 2 giant sets; 8 reps, 15 reps, 20 reps
Leg Curl: 2 giant sets; 8 reps, 15 reps, 20 reps
Calf Raises: 2 giant sets; 8 reps, 15 reps, 20 reps

Week Nine: Day 2...Upper Body:
Dips: 3 giant sets; 6 reps, 10 reps, 12 reps
Seated Dumbbell Bicep Curl: 2 giant sets; 6 reps, 10 reps, 12 reps
Triceps Extensions: 3 giant sets; 6 reps, 10 reps, 12 reps
Seated Dumbbell Shoulder Press: 2 giant sets; 6 reps, 10 reps, 12 reps
Wide Grip Pull-Ups: 2 giant sets; 6 reps, 10 reps, 12 reps

Week Nine: Day 1, 2, 3...Abs:
Cable Crunches: 3 sets; 20 reps
Cable Oblique Crunches: 3 sets; 20 reps

Week Ten: Day 1 and 3...Legs:
Squats: 3 sets; 8 reps
Leg Extension: 3 sets; 8 reps
Leg Curl: 3 sets; 8 reps
Calf Raises: 3 sets; 8 reps

Week Ten: Day 2…Upper Body:
Bench Press: 3 sets; 8 reps
Seated Dumbbell Bicep Curl: 3 sets; 8 reps
Triceps Extensions: 3 sets; 8 reps
Seated Dumbbell Shoulder Press: 3 sets; 8 reps
Wide Grip Pull Downs: 3 sets; 8 reps

Week Ten: Day 1, 2, 3…Abs:
Cable Crunches: 3 sets; 25 reps
Cable Oblique Crunches: 3 sets; 25 reps

Week Eleven: Day 1 and 3…Legs:
Leg Press: 2 supersets; 10 reps, 20 reps
Leg Extension: 2 supersets; 10 reps, 20 reps
Leg Curl: 2 supersets; 10 reps, 20 reps
Calf Raises: 2 supersets; 10 reps, 20 reps

Week Eleven: Day 2…Upper Body:
Dips: 2 supersets; 8 reps, 10 reps
Seated Dumbbell Bicep Curl: 2 supersets; 8 reps, 10 reps
Triceps Extensions: 2 supersets; 8 reps, 12 reps
Seated Alternating Dumbbell Press: 2 supersets; 8 reps, 12 reps
Wide Grip Pull Downs: 2 supersets; 8 reps, 12 reps

Week Eleven: Day 1, 2, 3…Abs:
Cable Crunches: 4 sets; 20 reps
Cable Oblique Crunches: 4 sets; 20 reps

Week Twelve: Day 1 and 3…Legs:
Leg Press: 2 giant sets; 6 reps, 10 reps, 12 reps
Leg Extension: 2 giant sets; 6 reps, 10 reps, 12 reps
Leg Curl: 2 giant sets; 6 reps, 10 reps, 12 reps
Calf Raises: 2 giant sets; 6 reps, 10 reps, 12 reps

Week Twelve: Day 2…Upper Body:
Dips: 2 giant sets; 6 reps, 10 reps, 12 reps
Seated Dumbbell Bicep Curl: 2 giant sets; 6 reps, 10 reps, 12 reps
Triceps Extensions: 2 giant sets; 6 reps, 10 reps, 12 reps
Seated Dumbbell Shoulder Press: 2 giant sets; 6 reps, 10 reps, 12 reps
Wide Grip Pull-Ups: 2 giant sets; 6 reps, 10 reps, 12 reps

Week Twelve: Day 1, 2, 3...Abs:
Cable Crunches: 4 sets; 25 reps
Cable Oblique Crunches: 4 sets; 25 reps

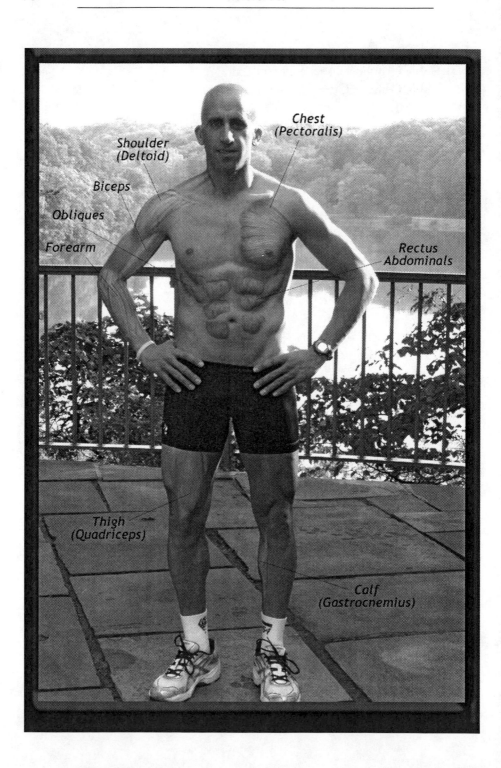

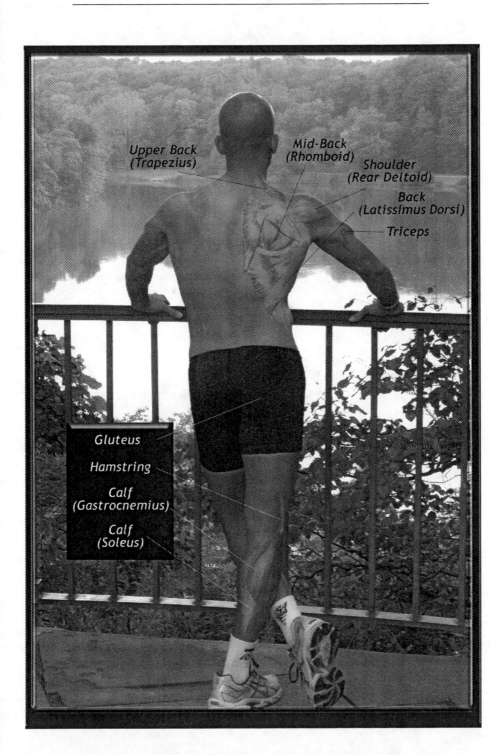

Upper Back
(Trapezius)

Mid-Back
(Rhomboid)

Shoulder
(Rear Deltoid)

Back
(Latissimus Dorsi)

Triceps

Gluteus

Hamstring

Calf
(Gastrocnemius)

Calf
(Soleus)

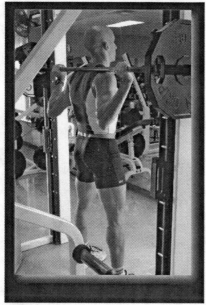

Smith Machine Squats

Be sure to rest the barbell on your upper back (trapezius muscle), not on your neck. Place your feet slightly wider than shoulder width apart. Slowly bend your knees, making sure your heels do not come off the ground.

Start

Do not go below parallel (your quadriceps [thigh] muscle will be parallel with the ground). In order to insure you do not go beyond parallel, adjust the safety spotters. The barbell will then hit the safety spotters when you have reached parallel. This exercise will train your gluteus maximus (buttocks) and your quadriceps muscles.

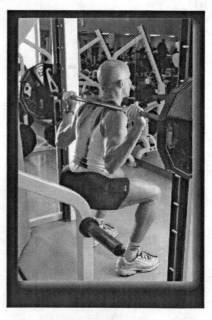

Finish

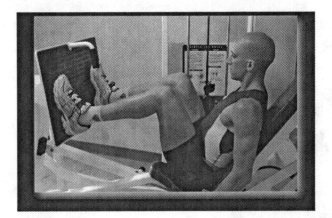

 Start with your knees bent, and place your feet on the platform slightly wider apart than shoulder width. Slowly extend your legs straight out. Be sure not to overextend your knees.

You want to maintain a slight bend in your knees. This exercise will train your gluteus maximus (buttocks) and your quadriceps (thighs).

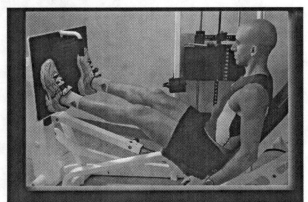

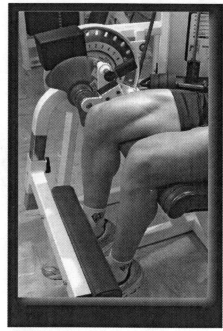

Leg Extensions

Start with your knees bent.

Start

Slowly extend your legs until they are straight. Be sure not to raise your hips off of the seat. Having to do so is a sign that the weight is too heavy. This exercise will train the quadriceps (thighs).

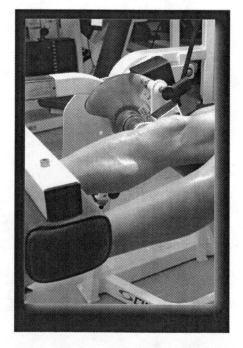

Finish

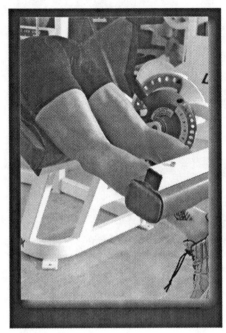

Leg Curl

Lie on your stomach, with the back of your lower leg on the pad of the machine. Slowly bring the weight toward your buttocks.

Be sure not to raise your hips off of the seat. Having to do so is a sign that the weight is too heavy. This exercise will train your hamstring muscles (upper leg).

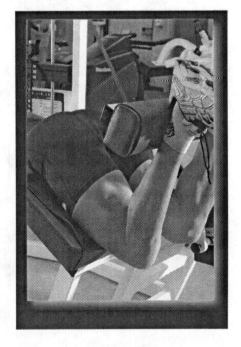

Finish

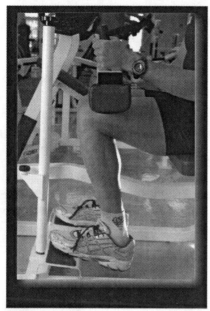

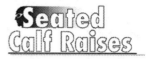

Keep the balls of your feet on the platform. Start by lowering your heals toward the floor.

Slowly raise the weight as though you are standing on your toes. You will perform this in the same manner as the standing calf raises. This exercise will train your calf muscles

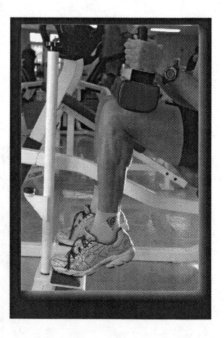

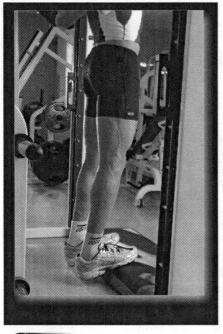

Start

Standing Calf Raises

Use the same machine as you did with the Smith Machine squats. Place the balls of your feet on a board that is 2 to 4 inches high. Starts with your heels as close to the ground as possible.

You will slowly raise yourself, now standing on your toes. This exercise will train your calf muscles.

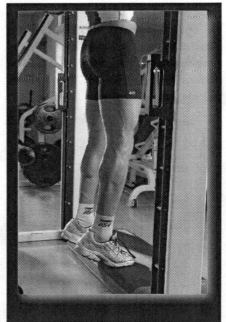
Finish

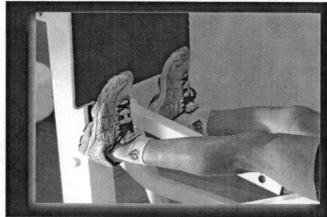

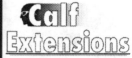

You will use the same machine as you did with the leg press. Place only the balls of your feet on the platform, slightly wider than shoulder width. Slowly extend your legs. Be sure to maintain a slight bend in your knees.

With your legs extended, slowly allow the platform to bring your toes closer to you, and then extend your feet as though you were standing on your toes. This exercise will train your calves (lower legs).

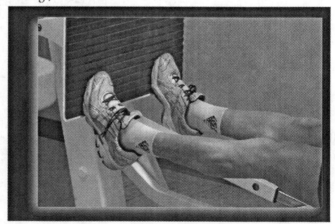

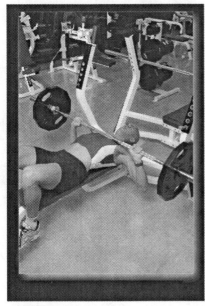

Flat Bench Press

Use a grip that is slightly wider than shoulder width. Slowly bring the barbell down to the middle of your chest, and extend your arms back up.

Do not bounce the barbell off of your chest. Having to do so is a sign that the weight is too heavy. This exercise will train your pectoral muscles (chest).

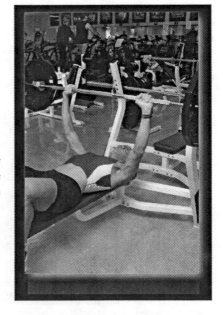

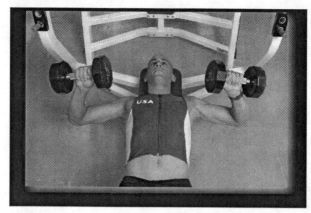

Flat Bench Dumbbell Press

Start   Start with the dumbbells at the side of your chest. Your arms should make a 90° angle.

Slowly raise the dumbbells straight up until they touch. Then slowly lower the dumbbells and repeat. This exercise will train your pectoral muscles (chest).

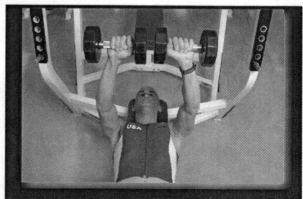

Finish

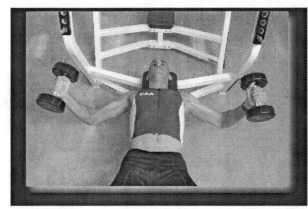

Flat Bench Dumbbell Fly

Start

Start with a slight bend in your elbows. You will maintain this bend in your elbows throughout the exercise.

Imagine having a small barrel on your chest. You will now bring the dumbbells up as though you were wrapping them around a barrel. This exercise will train your pectoral muscles (chest)

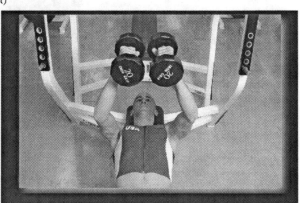

Finish

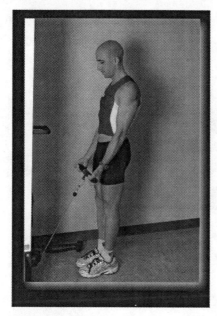

Straight Bar Bicep Curl

Be sure to keep your elbows in, and do not arch your back when performing the bicep curl.

Start

If you are arching your back, the weight is too heavy, and you are not isolating your biceps. This exercise will train your biceps.

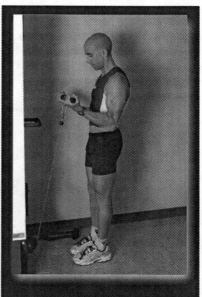

Finish

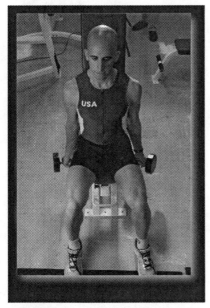

Seated Dumbbell Bicep Curl

Start with both dumbbells at your side. Be sure to keep you back against the bench. This will keep you from "cheating" and will isolate your biceps muscles.

Start

Slowly raise one dumbbell at a time, and then lower to the starting position. You will then repeat this same motion with the other arm. This exercise will train your biceps muscle.

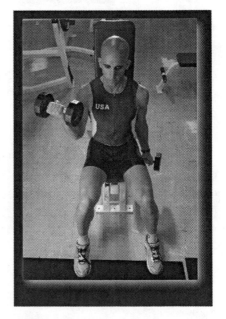

Finish

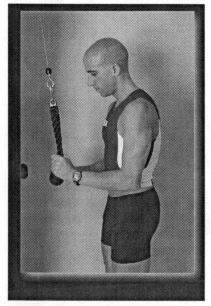

Start with your arms at a 90° angle.

Slowly extend your arms. Always maintain a slight bend in your elbows. Return your arms to the 90° angle (do not let the arms bend more than 90°). This exercise will train your triceps (back of upper arm).

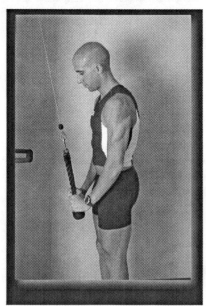

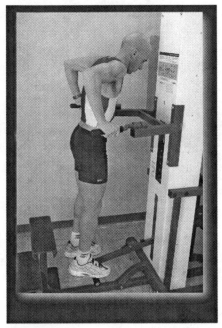

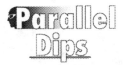

Parallel Dips

Place your hands on the side bars, and step onto the platform, allowing your body to drop. Start with your arms at a 90° angle.

Slowly extend your arms. Be sure not to overextend them. Always maintain a slight bend in your elbows. This exercise will train your triceps (back of upper arm), deltoids (shoulders), and pectoral muscles (chest).

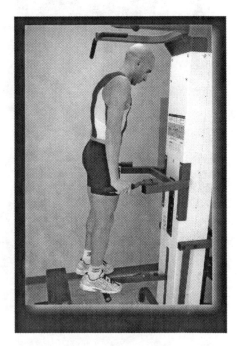

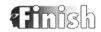

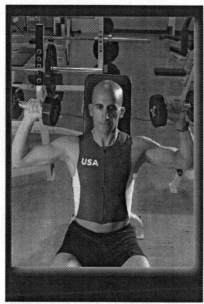

Seated Dumbbell Shoulder Press

Start with the dumbbells at your side, and make sure that your arms are at a 90° angle.

Start

Slowly raise the dumbbells above your head until the dumbbells touch. Do not fully extend your arms, and keep a slight bend in your elbows. This exercise will work your deltoids (shoulders).

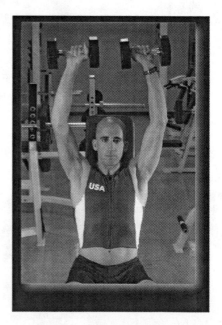

Finish

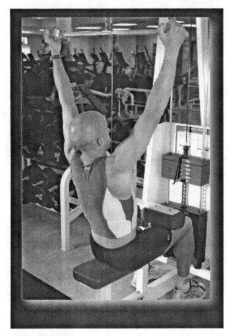

Wide-grip Pull Down

Start with your arms extended above your head. Slowly bring the bar toward your chest. The key is not to rock your upper body to bring the weight down. This is a sign that the weight is too heavy.

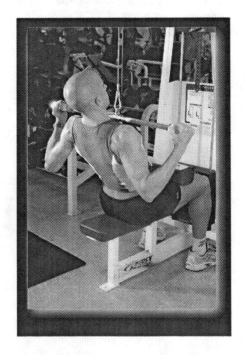

You want to bring the bar toward your upper-middle chest. To ensure you are working the proper muscles, you want to bring your chest forward and roll your shoulders back, as though you are bringing your shoulder blades together. You should feel this working your back. This exercise will work your latissimus dorsi (back muscle).

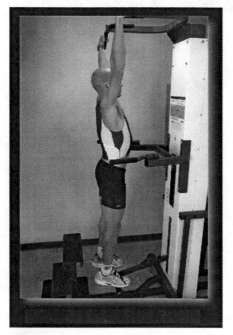

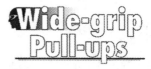

Grab the overhead bar with as wide a grip as possible. Step onto the platform, and let your arms extend fully so that you are hanging.

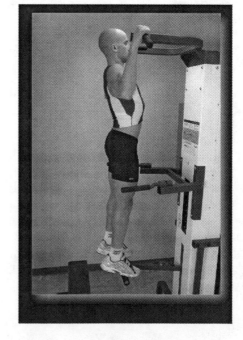

Slowly pull yourself up. This exercise will train your latissimus dorsi (back muscle).

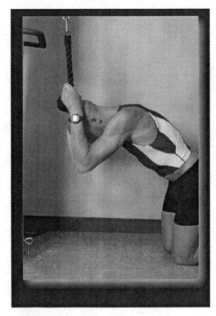

Abdominal Cable Crunch

To isolate your abdominal muscles, be sure to rest your hands on your head. Do not use your upper body to perform the abdominal crunch.

Start

Be sure to use only your abdominal muscles to perform this exercise. This exercise will train the rectus (front) abdominal muscles.

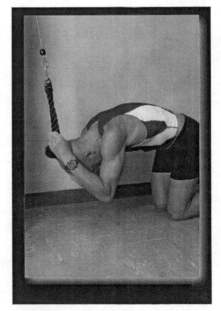

Finish

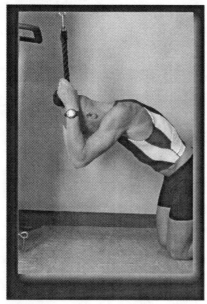

Abdominal Cable Oblique Crunch

You will use the same starting position as the abdominal cable crunch.

Start

Instead of crunching straight down, bring your elbow toward the opposite knee. Be sure not to use your upper body to perform this exercise. This exercise will train the oblique (side) abdominal muscles.

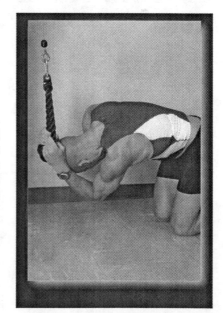

Finish

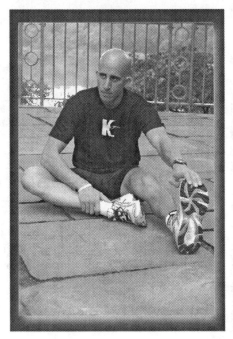

Hamstring Stretches

Be sure to keep a slight bend in the knee of the extended leg. The farther you lean toward your extended leg, the more you will stretch the hamstring. Repeat this with the other leg. Hold the stretch for approximately 10 seconds.

Place you leg on a structure approximately knee high. Keep a slight bend in your knee. Slowly reach toward your toe until you feel a slight stretch in your hamstring. Repeat this for the other leg. Hold this stretch for approximately 10 seconds.

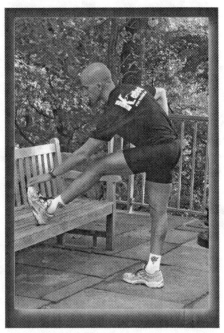

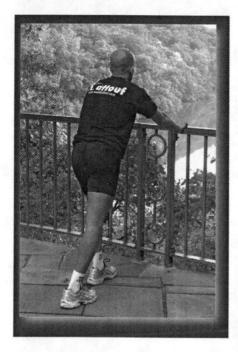

Calf
(gastrocnemius)
Stretch

Place one leg in front of the other. This exercise stretches the calf of the back leg in this position. Keep the heel of this leg on the ground. Slowly lean forward until you feel a slight stretch in your calf. Repeat this for the other leg. Hold the stretch for approximately 10 seconds.

Calf
(soleus)
Stretch

Perform this in the same way as the previous stretch, but bend the knee of your back leg. Repeat this for the other leg. This will allow you to stretch the smaller calf (soleus) muscle. Hold this stretch for approximately 10 seconds.

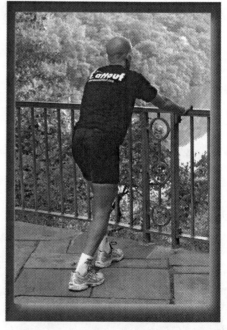

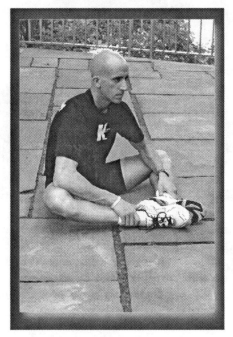

Adductor
(inner thigh)
Stretches

Hold your ankles, and with your elbows, gently press you knees toward the ground. Hold the stretch for approximately 10 seconds.

Slowly lean to one side until you feel a stretch in your adductor. Repeat this for the other leg. Hold this stretch for approximately 10 seconds.

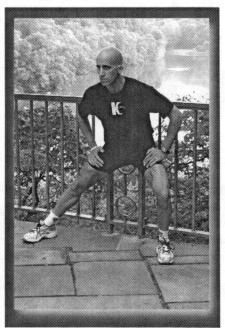

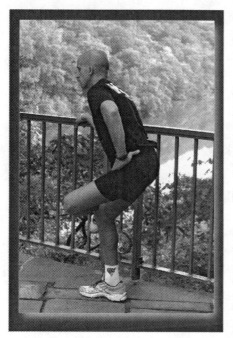

Hip/ Gluteus Stretch

Cross one leg over the other. Slowly bend you knee as though you are sitting in a chair. You should feel a stretch in your hip and gluteus. Repeat this for the other leg. Hold the stretch for approximately 10 seconds.

Hip Flexor Stretch

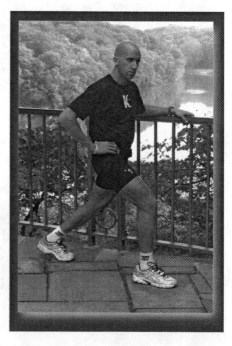

Place one leg behind the other. Bend your front knee while keeping the back leg straight. Slowly lean forward until you feel a stretch in the hip flexor of your back leg. Repeat this for the other leg. Hold this stretch for approximately 10 seconds.

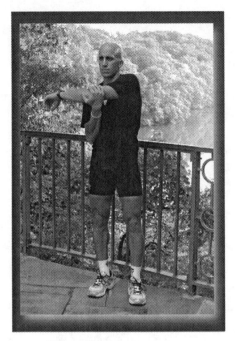

Rear Shoulder (deltoid) Stretch

Cross one arm over your chest. With your other hand, hold the elbow of the arm that is across your chest. Slowly pull on your elbow until you feel a stretch in your rear deltoid. Repeat this for the other arm. Hold the stretch for approximately 10 seconds.

Thigh (quadriceps) Stretch

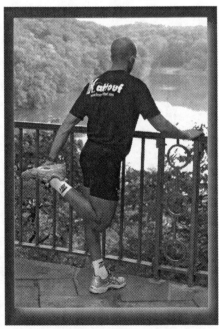

Hold one foot with the opposite hand. This will cause less stress on the inside of your knee. Slowly pull on your foot until you feel a stretch in your thigh. Repeat this for the other leg. Hold this stretch for approximately 10 seconds.

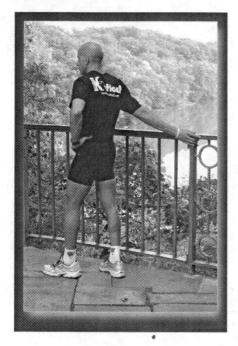

Chest
(pectoralis)
Stretch

Place your arm against a wall or something similar. Slowly rotate your body away from the wall until you feel a slight stretch in your chest. Repeat this for the other arm Hold the stretch for approximately 10 seconds.

Triceps
Stretch

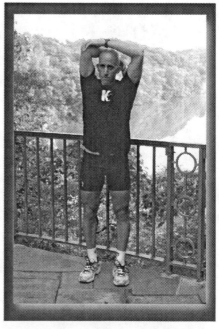

Place one arm above your head, and bend your elbow so that your hand is behind your head. Grab your elbow with your other hand. Slowly pull on your elbow until you feel a slight stretch in your triceps. Hold this stretch for approximately 10 seconds.

Fitness and Cardiovascular Program

Essentially, there are two ways to perform cardiovascular exercise. High intensity is considered anaerobic training, and lower intensity is referred to as aerobic training. The majority of your training will be aerobic. This aerobic training, combined with your weight training and your nutrition program, will give you all the necessary tools to achieve optimum fitness.

The majority of individuals I have trained over the years came from a background of too much intensity too often in their cardiovascular training. Let's look at this all too common scenario: An individual begins a fitness program in order to lose weight. Their training volume and intensity increases each week. As the weeks progress, they begin to get frustrated and lose motivation due to increased exercise but little or no weight loss. Does this sound familiar?

105

What happened here? The reason this individual could not lose weight even though they were exercising more is a combination of two factors: (1) Most likely they were exercising at too high of an intensity. (2) Their nutrition did not complement their increase in exercise. Remember what I said earlier…you must eat in order to lose weight.

Your cardiovascular program will be designed strictly around your heart rate. Your heart is your body's barometer; therefore, a heart rate monitor will be critical for your program. A heart rate monitor consists of a chest strap and a watch. The electrodes on the chest strap read your heart rate (for more information on heart rate monitors, refer to Chapter 13). This is like having a coach (me) on your wrist. Your heart rate will determine your exercise intensity. Just as the number of repetitions in your weight training determines how much weight to lift, your heart rate will determine how fast or slow you need to exercise. Beginners will find that they will have to go slow on the treadmill, exercise bike, and so forth to keep their heart rate in its prescribed heart rate zone. Those more advanced will be able to push the pace a bit without going above their heart rate zone.

As you progress through this program, you will find that you can walk, jog, ride, and so on faster at a lower heart rate. For example, let's say you have to walk at 3.5 mph on a treadmill during the first week in order to keep your heart rate in the proper zone. By week three and four, you will be able to walk at 4–4.5 mph at the same heart rate. This is a great sign of improved fitness…being able to go faster at the same heart rate. I mentioned earlier that in the past you might have associated weight training with building big muscles. Along similar lines, you may be of the attitude that in order to get a great cardiovascular workout, you must feel exhausted when you are finished. If so, you are not alone. I teach a lot of spinning classes (indoor cycling) and this is the attitude of the majority of those in my spin classes. Just as I have changed their view of cardiovascular training with the use of heart rate monitors, yours will change as well. As long as you are training in the prescribed heart rate zones, you are on your path to optimum fitness. Without a heart rate monitor, it is very difficult to judge how easy or hard to work out. You can follow a very subjective scale of perceived effort. This scale is based on a 0–10 perceived effort. Zero is considered minimal effort while a ten is maximal effort. The difficulty is correlating your heart rate with your perceived effort. Most people underestimate their perceived effort, which usually translates into a higher than prescribed exercise heart rate. Train with a heart rate monitor, follow your heart, and all of the guesswork will be eliminated. This will make your cardiovascular program very easy to follow.

Determining your heart rate zones (Refer to the charts on the following pages):

The following is an example for a fifty-year-old individual. Please, do not worry; you will not have to figure out each heart rate zone for yourself. The charts on the following pages will give you each heart rate zone based on your age. I am providing the formula for you in order to understand where these heart rate numbers come from.

- **220 - your age = maximum heart rate**
- 220 - 50 (years old) = 170 (maximum heart rate)

- *Seven heart rate zones:*
  Based off of a percentage of your maximum heart rate
- Level 1: 60% of your maximum $170 \times .60 = 102$ beats per minute (BPM)
- Level 2: 65% of your maximum $170 \times .65 = 110$ BPM
- Level 3: 70% of your maximum $170 \times .70 = 119$ BPM
- Level 4: 75% of your maximum $170 \times .75 = 128$ BPM
- Level 5: 80% of your maximum $170 \times .80 = 136$ BPM
- Level 6: 85% of your maximum $170 \times .85 = 145$ BPM
- Level 7: 90% of your maximum $170 \times .90 = 153$ BPM

To determine your prescribed heart rates, find your age along the left side of the following charts. Once you find your age, find the column along the top of the chart for your prescribed heart rate percentage for your workout. Match this column with the row associated with your age and this is the heart rate at which is prescribed for your cardiovascular workout.

Heart Rate Zone

AGE	65%	70%	75%	80%	85%	90%	Max
14	134	144	155	165	175	185	206
15	133	144	154	164	174	185	205
16	133	143	153	163	173	184	204
17	132	142	152	162	173	183	203
18	131	141	152	162	172	182	202
19	131	141	151	161	171	181	201
20	130	140	150	160	170	180	200
21	129	139	149	159	169	179	199
22	129	139	149	158	168	178	198
23	128	138	148	158	167	177	197
24	127	137	147	157	167	176	196
25	127	137	146	156	166	176	195
26	126	136	146	155	165	175	194
27	125	135	145	154	164	174	193
28	125	134	144	154	163	173	192
29	124	134	143	153	162	172	191
30	124	133	143	152	162	171	190
31	123	132	142	151	161	170	189
32	122	132	141	150	160	169	188
33	122	131	140	150	159	168	187
34	121	130	140	149	158	167	186
35	120	130	139	148	157	167	185
36	120	129	138	147	156	166	184
37	119	128	137	146	156	165	183
38	118	127	137	146	155	164	182
39	118	127	136	145	154	163	181
40	117	126	135	144	153	162	180
41	116	125	134	143	152	161	179
42	116	125	134	142	151	160	178
43	115	124	133	142	150	159	177
44	114	123	132	141	150	158	176
45	114	123	131	140	149	158	175
46	113	122	131	139	148	157	174
47	112	121	130	138	147	156	173
48	112	120	129	138	146	155	172
49	111	120	128	137	145	154	171
50	111	119	128	136	145	153	170

Heart Rate Zone

AGE	65%	70%	75%	80%	85%	90%	Max
51	110	118	127	135	144	152	169
52	109	118	126	134	143	151	168
53	109	117	125	134	142	150	167
54	108	116	125	133	141	149	166
55	107	116	124	132	140	149	165
56	107	115	123	131	139	148	164
57	106	114	122	130	139	147	163
58	105	113	122	130	138	146	162
59	105	113	121	129	137	145	161
60	104	112	120	128	136	144	160
61	103	111	119	127	135	143	159
62	103	111	119	126	134	142	158
63	102	110	118	126	133	141	157
64	101	109	117	125	133	140	156
65	101	109	116	124	132	140	155
66	100	108	116	123	131	139	154
67	99	107	115	122	130	138	153
68	99	106	114	122	129	137	152
69	98	106	113	121	128	136	151
70	98	105	113	120	128	135	150
71	97	104	112	119	127	134	149
72	96	104	111	118	126	133	148
73	96	103	110	117	125	132	147
74	95	102	110	116	124	131	146
75	94	102	109	115	123	131	145
76	94	101	108	114	122	130	144
77	93	100	107	114	122	129	143
78	92	99	107	143	121	128	142
79	92	99	106	113	120	127	141
80	91	98	105	112	119	126	140
81	90	97	104	111	118	125	139
82	90	97	104	110	117	124	138
83	89	96	103	110	116	123	137
84	88	95	102	109	116	122	136
85	88	95	101	108	115	122	135
86	87	94	101	107	114	121	134

Cardiovascular Exercise Tips

- **Consult your physician prior to starting your fitness program.**

- Refer to the heart rate monitor charts on the preceding pages to find your age and prescribed heart rate percentage.

- Your cardiovascular program is based on two days per week, with an optional third day if you choose to do additional cardiovascular training.

- Be sure to stretch (refer to the photo-instruction in Chapter 11) before and after working out. It is more important to stretch following your workout than prior to it.

- For each cardiovascular workout, be sure to warm up and warm down for five minutes. The warm up and warm down will be performed below 65% of your maximum heart rate (refer to heart rate zone charts on the preceding pages). For example, during week one on your weight training days: warm up below 65% of your maximum heart rate for five minutes, work out for ten minutes at 65–75% of your maximum heart rate, warm down for five minutes below 65% of your maximum heart rate. This will total your twenty minutes.

- **Fitness Test Guidelines:** Be sure to perform your fitness test on either a treadmill or a stationary bike. It is important to keep it consistent each time. If you choose the treadmill, use the treadmill for each fitness test. Following each test, record the total distance covered, average heart rate, max heart rate, maximum speed, and ending speed. Over the twelve weeks, you can compare your fitness tests and watch your overall fitness improve.

- Following week twelve, repeat the fitness program from week one. This will keep you from overtraining. Once you repeat week one, you will find an increased level of fitness; therefore, you will find yourself going faster at these lower heart rate levels. Once you begin to repeat week one, the one aspect you want to alter is your total training time. Keep the minimum cardiovascular time to thirty minutes. For example, repeating week one, train for a minimum of thirty minutes on both the weight training and non-weight training days at 65–70% of your max heart rate.

Week 1:	
Weight training days	20 min @ 65–70% of max hr
Non-weight training day	25 min @ 65–70% of max hr
Optional	25 min @ 65–70% of max hr
Week 2:	
Weight training days	25 min @ 65–70% of max hr
Non-weight training day	30 min @ 65–70% of max hr
Optional	30 min @ 65–70% of max hr
Week 3: Fitness Test	
Weight training days	30 min @ 65–70% of max hr
Non-weight training day	**Fitness Test:** 30 min @ 75–80% of max hr. Prior to fitness test, warm up for 5 min and following fitness test, warm down for 5 min.
Optional	25 min @ 65–70% of max hr
Week 4:	
Weight-training days	30 min @ 70–75% of max hr
Non-weight training day	30 min @ 70–75% of max hr
Optional	30 min @ 70–75% of max hr
Week 5:	
Weight training days	30–35 min @ 70–75% of max hr
Non-weight training day	35 min @ 70–75% of max hr
Optional	30–35 min @ 70–75% of max hr

Week 6: Fitness Test	
Weight training days	30–35 min @ 70–75% of max hr
Non-weight training day	**Fitness Test:** 30 min @ 75–80% of max hr. Be sure to include 5-minute warm-up and cooldown.
Optional	30–40 min @ 70–75% of max hr
Week 7:	
Weight training day	30–35 min @ 75–80% of max hr
Non-weight training day	40 min @ 75–80% of max hr
Optional	30–40 min @ 75–80% of max hr
Week 8:	
Weight training days	30–35 min @ 75–80% of max hr
Non-weight training day	45 min @ 75–80% of max hr
Optional	35–45 min @ 75–80% of max hr
Week 9: Fitness Test	
Weight training days	30–35 min @ 75–80% of max hr
Non-weight training day	**Fitness Test:** 30 min @ 75–80% of max hr. Be sure to include 5-minute warm-up and cooldown.
Optional	40–50 min (30 min @ 75–80% of max hr, 10–20 min @ 80–85% of max hr)
Week 10:	
Weight training days	30–35 min @ 80–85% of max hr
Non-weight training day	45 min (20 min @ 75–80% of max hr, 25 min @ 80–85% of max hr)
Optional	45–55 min (30 min @ 75–80% of max hr, 15–25 min @ 80–85% of max hr)

Week 11:	
Weight training days	30–35 min @ 80–85% of max hr
Non-weight training day	50 min (30 min @ 75–80% of max hr, 20 min @ 80–85% of max hr)
Optional	50–60 min (35 min @ 75–80% of max hr, 15–25 min @ 80–85% of max hr)
Week 12: Fitness Test	
Weight training days	30–35 min @ 80–85% of max hr
Non-weight training day	**Fitness Test:** 30 min @ 75–80% of max hr. Increase your warm-up and cooldown time to 10 minutes.
Optional	60 min (20 min @ 75–80% of max hr, 40 min @ 80–85% of max hr)

Recommended Fitness Equipment

The most important purchase you will make before you begin your life plan to achieve optimum fitness is a heart rate monitor (HRM). This will include a chest strap and a watch. Your HRM will serve as your coach on your wrist. Your heart is your body's barometer. It will tell you if you are training too hard or too easy. Listen to your heart and results will follow!

As for fitness equipment, if you belong to a fitness center, you will have access to treadmills, exercise bikes, ellipticals, stair steppers, indoor cycling classes, weight machines, dumbbells, and so forth. Now, if you are like a lot of individuals, you do not like to work out at a fitness center. You find comfort in working out at home. This can also be a huge time savings. For many people, the travel time alone to and from the fitness center can be your workout time.

Individuals with young children may find it much more convenient, as well as a necessity, to work out at home. So, if you are busy with family commitments, work, and other time commitments, how do you begin *Forever Fit?* Not to worry, because with minimal investment, you can have all the necessary equipment at home. Keep in mind, as previously mentioned, Forever Fit is a life plan. An easy-to-follow program you can continue to use and benefit from. For a lifetime of mental and physical well-being, your fitness equipment purchase will be well worth it. (As with the great nutritional products mentioned earlier, several fitness products listed here sponsor my athletic competitions. My clients and I have found them to provide superior results. But don't just take our word for it; try them yourself and see if they'll work for you!)

Heart rate monitor: This will be your best investment. A heart rate monitor (HRM) consists of a chest strap worn at the bottom of your sternum (chest bone) and a watch. These vary from the basic model that will simply read your heart rate to the high end that will also give you speed, distance, calories burned, max and average heart rate, audible alarm if you are outside of your prescribed heart rate zone, and many other features. I feel it is valuable to purchase an HRM that will give you your average heart rate. This will allow you to give yourself direct feedback when you perform the prescribed fitness tests. Some heart rate monitors also have downloadable capabilities. This enables you to save all of your training data and compare. Whether you buy the most basic or the most advanced, the important aspect is to stay within the prescribed heart rate zones. For a variety of makes and models, you can search "heart rate monitors" online.

Treadmill: If you enjoy walking, jogging, or running, a treadmill is for you. There are a lot of great home treadmills available. Depending on how high tech you are will determine what you buy. If you are a minimalist, the basic treadmill will do. If you want for more, you can purchase treadmills with pre-programmed workouts, heart rate monitor chips built in, downloadable courses from the Internet, and so forth. It is nice to have a treadmill that allows for small increment changes in both speed and incline. I highly suggest testing a few out in the fitness equipment store before finalizing your purchase. For a variety of makes and models, you can search "treadmills" online.

Exercise bike: If cycling is your passion, you have a plethora of styles and models available. As with the treadmills, you can go from extremely basic to very high tech. Exercise bikes are available with preprogrammed courses and heart rate monitor chips built in. If you enjoy indoor cycling classes, these bikes are also available for home use. This type of bike allows the rider to make numerous adjustments, making the workout as comfortable as possible. Most exercise bikes only allow for seat height adjustment. Bikes that are used in indoor cycling classes allow for seat height, fore and aft, and handlebar height adjustment. I feel you will get a great workout on either style. Enjoy your ride! For a variety of makes and models, you can search "exercise bikes" or "stationary bikes" online.

Stationary bike trainer: OK, so you have your own bike. It could be a road bike, mountain bike, or hybrid bike. Well, you are in luck. You can turn your bike into a stationary bike. If you live in areas in the country where riding outdoors year-round is next to impossible, a stationary bike trainer is a must. Your front wheel remains stationary while your rear wheel sits in the trainer. As you pedal, your rear wheel stays in motion, simulating riding on the road. I suggest buying the trainer that is as quiet as possible. You can visit your local bike shop for a variety of makes and models.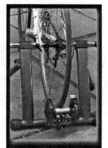

Weight machine: Various weight machines are made that will allow you to work out your entire body. These multiunits are created to take up as little space as possible. I have used a number of these units and they definitely get the job done. From bench press to squats and everything in between, none of your muscles will be left out. Some models use a weight stack while others use rods, bands, and so forth for resistance. I feel that you will get good quality resistance training no matter which style you choose. For a variety of makes and models, visit your local fitness equipment store or sporting goods store. You can also search "fitness equipment" online.

Dumbbells and bench: For a very cost-effective and space-saving weight training modality, here is your answer. With a few dumbbells and a multiposition bench, the majority of the prescribed exercises can be completed. Be sure to purchase a bench that will go from flat to upright. The amount of weight you buy is determined by your strength. Purchasing 3–4 different sets should be sufficient. The most effective dumbbell system is one that contains only two dumbbells but allows you to have weights varying from 5 lbs up to 90+ lbs. A simple pin and a quick change allow you to go from a 10 lb dumbbell to a 25 lb dumbbell. If you want to save space, this is for you. For a variety of dumbbells, visit your local fitness equipment store or sporting goods store.

PowerCranks: Whether you are a casual or avid cyclist, a runner, or you just want to improve your fitness, Power-Cranks can help get you there. If you thought you knew how to pedal a bike, think again. If you own a bike, you know your cranks arms are 180 degrees from one another. Well, not with PowerCranks. The crank arms both fall toward the ground; therefore, while pedaling, you are forced to pull up during your pedal stroke or you are not moving. Power-Cranks are the first (and only) devices that train the hip flex-ors and hamstring muscles and improve unconscious coordination ability. I have seen great results with mine. My leg strength has improved as well as my race performances. I recommend them not only to cyclists but to anyone look-ing to take their fitness to the next level. For more information on Power-Cranks, visit www.TeamKattouf.com and click on sponsors. Turn to Appendix A for ordering information.

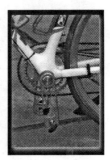

Rudy Project Eyewear: One unique aspect of Rudy Project Eyewear is their interchangeable lenses. Depending on the weather conditions, you can use a lens that is smoke, red, yellow, orange, and so forth. If you walk, jog, bike, or simply like the outdoors, Rudy Project Eyewear is for you. You will look and feel good in these technically cool eyewear. With various styles and colors, you will definitely find a pair that fits your style. With lenses that provide ultravio-let coating, you will protect your eyes from harmful UV rays that can cause various ocular problems. I like to show my patriotism when I race the world championships and wear my red, white, and blue Rudy's. Turn to Appendix A for ordering information.

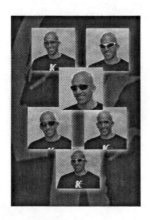

Section IV:
Putting It All Together

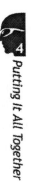

The First Day of the Rest of Your Life

Now it is time to put together everything that you have just read into an easy-to-follow, step-by-step life plan. Let's summarize your path to achieving optimum fitness and becoming forever fit into six easy-to-follow steps. This will allow you to see your entire plan come to life right in front of your eyes. You will repeat several of the steps that you have already completed in earlier chapters, but that's intentional. Repeating and reasserting your goals will reinforce your path to optimum fitness, and, if you find that your goals have changed or grown with the information you've learned in this book, it's OK to update them here.

Step number one: Rewrite the answers to the questions in Chapter 2.

1.   Why did you choose to read this book?

2.   What is your personal definition of optimum fitness?

Step number two: Write down your goal-dreams, positive thoughts, and successful moments. Be sure to share your goal-dreams with your support group.

1.   1 week:

2.   1 month:

3.   3 months:

4.   6 months:

5.   1 year:

6.   Positive thought #1:

7.   Positive thought #2:

8.   Successful moment #1:

9.　Successful moment #2:

10.　Successful moment #3:

Step number three: Weigh yourself, measure your body fat percentage, take your body measurements, and take photographs of yourself:

Body weight =
Body fat percentage =

1.　Neck:

2.　Chest:

3.　Upper arm:

4.　Waist (at level of navel):

5.　Hips:

6.　Upper thigh:

7.　Lower leg (calf):

8.　Photographs: YES or NO

Step number four: Design your nutrition plan. Using the chart in Chapter 8, design your nutrition for tomorrow. That soon, you ask? Absolutely! If you are waiting for a knock at your door to lead you to optimum fitness, you will probably be waiting a long time. No life changes, especially of this magnitude, will happen without your complete involvement and motivation. And obviously achieving optimum fitness is close to your heart, or you wouldn't have made it this far in the book. So why wait to improve your diet when you can begin tomorrow? Be sure to write down what you plan to eat and then follow this up with what you actually ate. I recommend making photocopies of this chart. Recording your planned foods versus your actual foods will keep you focused, and focus brings results.

Step number five: Obtain a heart rate monitor.

Step number six: Decide whether you plan to work out at home or at a fitness center. Take a look at your daily schedule and determine whether it permits you to work out in the morning, afternoon, or evening. Determine which three days (and possibly a fourth optional day) that you will work out.

1. Circle one: Home Fitness Center

2. Circle one: Morning Afternoon Evening

3. Circle three or four: M T W TH F SA SU

Putting these six steps together was probably quite easy due to the fact that you had most of it written down from the earlier chapters. This allows you to view your life plan as a whole instead of in its separate parts. Every plan for success, no matter how overwhelming it might seem at first, is really a series of smaller, achievable steps. And by taking on this plan step by step, you're ensuring that you will meet your goals.

I am so excited for you to begin your journey to achieve optimum fitness. You are to be commended for making the necessary lifestyle changes that will lead to a healthier body and mind. Remember to be patient and have fun. Looking at these six steps together brings about an even stronger sense of accountability. You know you are ready to make a change. Become passionate about your life plan, and embrace the changes you are about to embark upon. Watch for and note the sense of balance that will soon enter your life. Enjoy its effects, and don't be afraid to document the changes in your life that balance will bring; if you encounter challenges on your path to optimum fitness, these notes of success will serve as powerful, personal motivation to charge through the hard times and continue with your plan.

When you encounter obstacles on your journey, stay focused; reiterate your goal-dreams, and this will keep you on the right path. Be sure to ask yourself each night before you go to sleep, "What did I do today to get one step closer to achieving my goal-dreams?" Visualize your past successful experiences, and, in your mind, replay the wonderful emotions you experienced at that time. Watch your body go through positive changes as your journey progresses. Keep a healthy mind and your body will follow. Your self-esteem, confidence, and happiness will soon be at an all-time high. Enjoy achieving optimum fitness as you become forever fit. Today is the first day of the rest of your life!

Section V:
People Just Like You

FAQs, Success Stories, and Testimonials

FAQ's

Over the past thirteen years, my clients have asked some very good questions regarding nutrition and fitness. In this chapter I will highlight the most frequently asked questions. I think you will find this section very useful. If your question is not answered, feel free to e-mail me at rick@rickkattouf.com. I look forward to hearing from you.

What happens if I make poor nutrition choices for a meal, a day, or even a week?

The key is to get back on track as soon as possible. Many people are of the philosophy that if they indulge, they can make it up by skipping meals. "I made poor food choices for dinner, so I will skip breakfast tomorrow to make up for it." As previously mentioned, skipping meals will slow down your

127

metabolism (see Chapter 7). Just get back to thinking carbohydrates, protein, and fats. Be sure to plan ahead for your daily nutrition. This will minimize the potential for poor food choices. Please do not beat yourself up for having a bad meal for a day, or even bad meals for a week. You are only human after all. The good sign is that you recognized your poor choices and you are ready to correct for them.

Can I "cheat" at all on Forever Fit *nutrition program?*

"Cheating" or eating foods not on *Forever Fit* is going to happen to most of you at one time or another. Eating "not so clean" foods can slow your progress. Weight loss and body fat loss will be altered. With that being said, here is my suggestion to you: If you are going to "cheat," pick a meal rather than an entire day. If your food choices are not so good for a meal as opposed to an entire day, you will be able to recover much easier. Also, try to have your "not so clean" food earlier in the day as opposed to late at night.

I feel as if I am following the nutrition, but I gained a few pounds in the first couple weeks. Is this common?

Yes, it is common to see a weight fluctuation when you begin. Think of it like resetting a thermostat. You have to reset your body's thermostat, and until it starts to recalibrate, your body weight may fluctuate. Patience is the key. Your body weight did not go on overnight; therefore it will not come off overnight. Once you start noticing weight loss and body fat loss, you will continue to progress in the right direction.

I followed a low-carbohydrate diet, and now, after following Forever Fit, *I feel bloated. Is this normal?*

Yes, this is a very common dynamic following a low-carbohydrate diet. Carbohydrates retain water. By cutting these out as you did, the weight you lost was merely water weight, not body fat. Now that you are incorporating carbohydrates into your nutrition, your body will start to retain water, hence the bloated feeling. The good news is that this is temporary. Following a low-carbohydrate diet, your body's metabolism was greatly slowed. Now, following *Forever Fit*, you have to teach your body to jumpstart your metabolism. This will occur by following the nutrition as prescribed.

What happens if I drink alcohol while following Forever Fit?

Alcohol falls into my category of empty calories or unusable calories. Alcohol, in moderation, will not allow you to maximize your weight loss and body fat loss. We have to make choices in life and endure the consequences that follow. Understanding that drinking alcohol may slow your progress is a decision you have to make.

What if I count beer as my carbohydrate?

As the above answer states, alcohol comprises unusable calories. Yes, beer does have carbohydrates, but it cannot be substituted for another carbohydrate if you want to see results.

Since I began following Forever Fit, *I have become much hungrier than before. Is this normal?*

Yes, not only is this normal, but this is a great sign! Your metabolism has just been jumpstarted—congratulations! Prior to working with me, clients tell me they were never hungry. Now, they find themselves hungry every couple hours. Keep it up; you are right on track.

I am busy at work all day and do not eat between lunch and dinner. When I get home for dinner, I am famished, and I want to eat everything. What should I do?

What happens here is that when we skip meals or snacks, we are in a hormonal imbalance; therefore, we start to crave "bad" foods. We want to anything that crosses our path. The number one solution is to try and plan better and have foods available (such as Baker's Breakfast Cookies or MET-2) to prevent this. We all know that in reality this will happen from time to time. So, here is what to do when you get home. The body is famished and needs to be satiated, quickly. Understand, even though you are craving "bad" foods, whether you eat fast food at this point or a *Forever Fit* meal, your body will be satiated. Make a good food choice right when you get home (do not graze around the kitchen); sit down, relax, and enjoy. Shortly, you will be satisfied, your blood sugar will stabilize, and your cravings will significantly lessen.

Following dinner, I am not hungry before I go to bed. Do I still need to eat the snack prior to bed?

This is a great question. The answer is no. Many people eat dinner fairly late; therefore, little time transpires between dinner and bedtime. If you are satiated before going to bed, consider it a successful nutrition day, rest well, and start your next day's nutrition off right.

If I have an allergy to peanuts. What can I do for my dietary fat?

I definitely do not want you to have an adverse reaction in this case. Heart-healthy vegetable oils will become one of your main sources of fat. Extra-virgin olive oil (EVOO) is the healthiest choice, but other smart options include safflower oil and flax oil. Remember, even though these are the healthiest sources of oil-based fat for your diet, use them sparingly; 2 tsp of oil will serve you well. You can use them on your salad, sandwich, or to sauté your vegetables. Cheese can also be used as a source of fat. Sprinkle cheese on your salad or put some on your sandwich. Low-fat cheese is best. Hummus also is a very good source of fat. I would suggest 1 tbsp of hummus.

When I am working out and following my heart rates, I feel like I am going very slowly to stay within my prescribed zones. Am I getting any benefits by going this slow?

It sounds like you are right on track. First off, good job staying within the prescribed heart rates. And yes, this is very normal. Your fitness level simply has a lot of room for improvement. As you progress, you will find that you can go faster than these same heart rates. You first have to go slow in order to get faster and fitter. Please do not let your slow pace discourage you. You are still getting benefits, even though you're going slowly. Keep in mind, your fitness test will show you that you are improving despite the slow workout pace. As long as you are in your prescribed zone, you are right on.

What if I am unable to reach the prescribed heart rates for a certain workout?

Not to worry—this will happen at some point in your training. If you are working out, and you cannot reach the prescribed heart rate zones, simply continue your workout at a lower heart rate zone. You are still getting a lot of benefit, even at a lower zone. This can happen for a number of reasons, such as fatigue or stress.

I have been following Forever Fit *for some time now, and feel I have a pretty good feel for my pace and heart rates. Lately I have noticed I am working less hard but my heart rate is much higher. Is this normal?*

A higher heart rate at a lower perceived effort can be a sign of many things. You may have a low-grade infection and could be on the verge of becoming sick (possibly with a cold or flu). I recommend taking a rest day or two and reevaluate. If it persists, take another day or so of rest, get plenty of sleep; you want to combat the potential illness. Other factors of higher than normal heart rates could be sleep deprivation and stress. Once again, these situations show that your heart is your body's barometer; be sure to listen to it.

I have a cold (or flu). I still want to work out, so what should I do?

If you have an upper respiratory infection (chest and head congestion), take a few days off from any cardiovascular exercise. Weight training at this time is acceptable. A lot of this depends on the severity of your symptoms. The key is not to do anything that will exacerbate your illness. When in doubt, rest! Once you begin feeling better, do not start working out too intense. For the days to follow, you will want to keep your heart rates about 5 to 10 beats per minute lower than prescribed until you feel one hundred percent better.

I have been following the Forever Fit *fitness program for a week, and I am sore. What should I do?*

Soreness, especially if you are new to working out is normal. Injuries are something we want to avoid like the plague, so taking a rest day would be highly suggested. Rest will help facilitate recovery. Keep in mind, your soreness, referred to as Delayed Onset Muscle Soreness (DOMS), may not appear for a day or two following a workout. Always be cautious and start with light weights as not to put too much stress on the muscles. Once you get stronger, you can slowly start to increase you weights.

I like to walk, run, and bike outdoors. Can I work out outdoors instead of on the treadmill or exercise bike?

Absolutely! Be aware that perceived effort and heart rates differ between a treadmill or exercise bike and outdoor training. The key is simply to follow the prescribed heart rates whether inside or outside.

As a walker (or runner), does it matter what shoes I wear?

Correct shoes are a big key to keeping injuries away. A true running shoe (not a "cross training" shoe) is critical. I highly suggest going to your local running store as opposed to a large national shoe store. Your local running store employees will have better knowledge to fit you with a shoe that suits your needs. Everyone has a different body type and a different gait; therefore, let your local running store evaluate and suggest what is best for you.

My typical lifting and cardiovascular workout takes me approximately 45 to 60 minutes to complete. What if I only have 20 to 30 minutes to work out? Should I skip the workout?

Keep this in mind: something is better than nothing. In this case, with limited time to work out, I suggest completing the prescribed weight training exercises. Hold off on the cardiovascular exercise, and maybe you will find time later in the week to make it up. This will allow you to maximize your allotted workout time. Time management is the key. Whatever available time you have, maximize it, and you will make yourself proud!

Success Stories

Over my thirteen years of nutrition and fitness coaching, I have worked with many unique individuals. As a coach, nothing is more satisfying than seeing my clients succeed. Everyone's goals and dreams are different, and this is what makes coaching so much fun. Watching one person after the next achieving their goals brings a smile to my face. I want to share some success stories with you. All names used in these stories are not the client's real names. I truly look forward to hearing from you and sharing in your success as I have with all of my clients. I welcome the smile that your story will put on my face!

As a twenty-year-old premed college student just starting my nutrition and fitness business, I was faced with my first challenge. Carrie, a very pleasant woman in her mid-twenties, approached me at the local fitness center. I saw

Carrie's motivation immediately. Fed up with being overweight, she was ready to make a change in her life. Carrie stood 5'8" and 315 pounds. She followed my lead and did not deviate. We met at the fitness center a few days per week. Carrie, from the start, followed the nutrition program as prescribed. After eighteen months Carrie was a new person. Her confidence was soaring and she wore the nicest smile from ear to ear. Carrie had lost an astounding 125 pounds! By following my lead, she lost an average of seven pounds of body fat per month (this translates into 1.75 pounds of body fat per week.). More impressive than the weight loss is that to this day Carrie has kept it off. Carrie definitely put a smile on my face.

John, forty-eight years old, contacted me regarding my coaching services. I could sense John's apprehension at first. He questioned if my heart rate training and nutrition program would allow him to reach his goals. At 6'1", 220 pounds, John was looking to become leaner, allowing him to become a better cyclist. John took to my program like a duck to water. John has always said that once he finally started my program, it just made sense to him. He liked its user-friendly nature. John is now a lean 189 pounds. This is a loss of thirty-one pounds. Johns body fat dropped from 26% (a male over 25% body fat is considered obese) to an unbelievable 10.5%. As John's coach, I could not be happier.

Mary, thirty-seven years old with two children, was interested in my coaching services. She was thin and fit, but was looking to take her running to the "next level." Mary had a goal to qualify for the Boston Marathon. Mary adopted the heart rate training and nutrition program and began to see results immediately. She could see her fitness level improving and her energy levels higher. Mary was able to test her fitness in a preparation running race. Somewhat skeptical about racing by heart rate, she stuck to the plan as prescribed. She turned in a top performance and never felt better in the days following the race. Following my nutrition and training plan, Mary was allowing her body to recover better than ever. With the qualifying marathon on the horizon, you will have to stay tuned. I feel good about this one!

Molly, a forty-eight-year-old mother of two and a very accomplished tri-athlete, called me after visiting my Web site. She inquired about my nutrition program. Molly wanted to take her training and racing to the next level and felt her nutrition needed some tweaking. I performed a nutrition analysis on Molly and found a few areas that she could improve. A coach herself, Molly was very coachable. She followed everything I prescribed. Molly noticed immediate changes, as she was able to reduce her body fat. Her energy levels were higher, making her training and racing that much better. She soon noticed less stomach distress while training. Molly had more energy during swimming, cycling, and running, and she was able to recover easier.

Dr. Bill, a thirty-six-year-old radiologist, approached me regarding my services. Bill had an extremely demanding schedule. He had noticed after years of medical school, residency, and so on that his physical activity had been brought to a standstill. His body weight had crept up to 176 pounds. Bill felt his nutrition was poor due to being in the hospital all day. He decided to hire me. I needed to prescribe a schedule for Bill that would complement his busy schedule. Following a nutrition analysis, I prescribed a nutrition plan for him. I taught Bill that no matter what he ate, he could make better food choices. Knowing what the hospital had to offer, I incorporated better foods for Bill to eat. He did his homework and followed the nutrition and fitness plan. Bill lost sixteen pounds and looked great. He was thrilled with his higher energy levels and leaner look. Bill continues to maintain his weight loss while improving his fitness level.

Sam, thirty-seven years old, contacted me after talking to a client of mine. Sam wanted to become leaner in order to improve his race results in triathlon. He is married, works full time, and has two children. After Sam's nutrition analysis, changes were implemented. Sam was very focused on the nutrition and fitness program. He instantly noticed increased energy levels. His triathlon performance was very good as well, taking thirty minutes off of his half-ironman time from the previous year. A half-ironman triathlon consists of a 1.2-mile swim, 56-mile bike, and 13.1-mile run. With a busy work and family schedule, Sam was somewhat limited in his time to train. He knew that if he stayed on course with the nutrition and fitness, results would follow; and that is exactly what he did. All season, Sam not only noticed faster race times, but also a better ability to recover. He was less sore following training and racing.

Roger, forty-three years old, approached me about my coaching services. Roger explained that he had surgery performed to reduce his weight. He said the surgery was successful, but he was stuck at the same body weight. Roger engaged in a low-intensity exercise program, and he could perform some cardiovascular machines for a maximum of twenty minutes. But despite this, Roger still weighed 380 pounds. After I explained my program to Roger, he hired me. He was very focused on both the nutrition and fitness program. Today, Roger can perform cardiovascular exercise for ninety minutes, quite an improvement from twenty minutes. After years of being stuck at 380 pounds, Roger is now 355 pounds and still losing.

Barry, thirty-two years old, received my coaching services as a birthday gift from his wife. His wife was a friend of a client of mine. Barry was ready for a change. His body weight was stuck at 200 pounds. He was an avid cyclist. Barry stuck to the prescribed program like glue. Instantly he noticed increased energy from the nutrition changes. Heart rate training was new to Barry. He saw how much better he felt following proper heart rates. In six short weeks, Barry lost ten pounds of body fat, improved his cycling performance, and greatly increased his everyday energy levels. After years of working out, cycling, and being stuck at his body weight, Barry was able to realize dramatic changes after only six short weeks of following my program.

Ben, a twenty-two-year-old golf pro, approached me regarding my services. He was referred to me from a former client. After meeting with Ben, he was extremely motivated to get started. Before beginning, I received a call from Ben. He said he was not ready to begin. After a few months passed, I got a second phone call—Ben said he was ready to begin. At 5'9" and 210 pounds and soon to be married, Ben wanted to lose weight. Ben was strict with his nutrition and training. Aside from the physical changes Ben desired, he felt his mental game needed work. I constantly worked with him on mental approaches that could turn him around. He followed my lead, lost twenty-five pounds, was refit for his tuxedo, and played the best golf round of his life.

My most favorite female client over my thirteen years is sixty-year-old Jackie…after all, she is my mother! At 46 years of age, my mom was ready for change. My mother was never heavy, but she also never worked out. One day the scale read a number that sent a shock through her veins. At 5'3", my mom hit 155 pounds. She was ready to work out and eat right. My mom, to this day, follows my lead. Today, at sixty years of age, she is leaner than ever. At 128 pounds, she is younger looking, more beautiful than ever, and often asked if she is my sister or girlfriend! Jackie is a living example that no matter what age you are, body weight and body fat loss are possible.

As not to top my most favorite female client, I have to introduce you to my most favorite male client. He is my best friend and just happens to be my father. As Mom did, Dad follows my lead as well. My father ran two marathons in his fifties. As a doctor and businessman, my father's schedule is extremely demanding. In and out of airports and hotels, it would be easy to make bad food choices. No matter what, my father finds time to work out and his food choices are right on. At sixty-one years old, he is leaner than ever. At 6' tall and 180 pounds, he is many times mistaken as my brother! Once again, nutrition and fitness goals can be attained at any age.

Testimonials

"I can only describe my experience with Rick as 'life altering.' As a busy trial attorney, I found myself subtly gaining weight as I approached forty. I have always trained hard and often, but seemed to be going in reverse. Rick then designed the most basic and easy-to-follow nutrition and exercise regimen for me, which introduced me to proper heart rate training and weight lifting. The nutrition plan he gave me was so easy to follow because it allowed for my favorite thing: eating…and eating often (the right foods, that is). After six months of Rick's tutelage, I have lost that extra 10 pounds and my energy and fitness levels have soared. Rick is a motivator extraordinaire and a walking fitness and nutrition encyclopedia. Thanks for everything, Rick!"

Robert I. Shaker
www.shakerlaw.com

"Well, we will keep it short and give the facts...My kids were out of school and on their own, so I decided it was time for me to get back into cycling, and I wanted to race. I needed someone to help me understand all the books I had been reading, which by this time had me completely confused! I then picked up Rick Kattouf's business card at the local fitness center. After reading all of Rick's qualifications, I felt he would be able to help me improve as an endurance athlete.

"I called Rick and set up an appointment. He explained his nutrition and fitness program. I still remember what he said that first day: 'If you hire me as your coach, give us both a fair chance. Follow my nutrition and fitness program for six weeks, and then you can decide if you want to continue.' When I began, I was 220 pounds and averaging 15–16 mph on the bike. After five months of coaching I lost 15% body fat and dropped to 190 pounds. I was much stronger and leaner, now averaging 19–22 mph. I decided in the spring to try running as well as compete in duathlons. I entered a seven race series (I am currently second in my age group 45–49).

"I have been more than pleased with Rick's training. He has taken me beyond the initial goals I had set for myself. (In fact, I surpassed all of my goals in my very first race by winning my age group!) I can honestly say that without Rick's training and nutrition program, I would not have accomplished half of what I have done so far!

"Remember, if you buy Rick's book or hire him for personal online coaching, give yourself a fair chance, follow his lead, and results will follow...believe me, it works!"

Rick Shreckengost

Learn to Fly
Channeled by E.A. Vicol

From hopes and fears to moments of speed
Rick I met to help my deed

First diet, then strength were the topics to share
When we spoke of the need to prepare

With pace and rhythm and a pat on the back
Rick and I plotted the course and track

Each form and task so carefully made
To support my goals with groundwork laid

And then the time for me comes near
I'll trust the plan sincere

My heart now beats with a quicken pace
Just a moment before the race

And in that moment I pause and wait
The way I've learned and the growth I've made

From a man that has shown
With a spark in his eye
That I, like him, can learn to fly

"Due to long hours of studying in medical school and thirty-six-hour shifts during four years of residency, I packed on twenty pounds that I just could not get rid of during the last ten years. Then I met Rick. He immediately designed a nutrition program that is healthy and practical to follow. At this point, I have learned to combine the proper food groups every time I eat without the need of looking at a list. This program really boosted my metabolism, which is a natural cause to gain weight as we get into our thirties…and beyond! Then he tailored a cardiovascular and weight training program based on realistic times per week (4) and time per day (1 hour) that I can be comfortable with. The results have been amazing; I've lost twenty-five pounds in five months and have kept it off even during times of not much ferrous discipline (you know what I mean!).

"I travel constantly, and what I like about Rick's plan is that he sends me a totally different program every Sunday evening via e-mail; I can be out of state or out of the country and all I have to do is print the program from the hotel's front desk and use their fitness facility. The fact that I can have a personal trainer without the hassles of missing an appointment and the affordable price makes this program truly unique and effective. I strongly endorse it to anybody!"

Sincerely,
Jorge E. Martinez-Llorens, MD
Board Certified Radiologist

"Running a marathon was my only goal, and luckily for me, I had the greatest coach to get me there. Finishing Chicago in 3:42 with no injury was the best feeling in the world. Rick's training program taught me so much about running the right way and how to run a race that you can actually feel great throughout the entire distance, which is very impressive to learn in preparation of any race. The best part of Rick's training program is his unbelievable knowledge about training and his confidence in your ability to achieve your goal. He is a great motivator and extremely supportive the entire way. It is amazing how quickly I converted to heart rate training and how effectively this training tool is used. Thank you so much, Rick, for your confidence in my running ability and your positive attitude throughout my entire training! For my first marathon, I definitely learned so much from you, and I knew that I was both mentally and physically ready to run with all your support!"

Lori Zelenak

"In the past eleven weeks, I lost fifteen pounds, got hooked on a new sport, made new friends, bought the fastest bike I will ever own, and impressed my son…all because of my association with you. Picking up your business card and calling was the healthiest thing I've done for myself (and family) in years!"

Todd Huna

"Let Rick take all the guesswork out of training and nutrition. There are so many books on how to train and eat; it is mind-boggling. I bought the books, tried to train myself and got nowhere!

"First you need to know a little about myself; I am short, overweight, and a cancer survivor.

"I got back into running, did my 5K in July 2002, and was happy to finish, albeit in last place. After the race, I was coaxed into running a marathon in the spring of 2003. I knew if I was going to finish, I was going to need some help. I met Rick at the gym and knew of his accomplishments. After reviewing my goals, Rick put together a very easy training and nutrition plan for me to follow. I work long hours and travel a lot, but with Rick's plan, I was able to follow it both at home and on the road.

"Well, ten months and thirty pounds later, I finished that marathon and I ran the same 5K, taking off over eight minutes from the previous year! I figured since I was in shape, I would try my hand in duathlons. Rick easily tailored my training for it. I had a great time and took second in the XL division. Rick and I concentrated on training for duathlons. (Duathlons consist of a 6.2-mile run, 24.8-mile bike, and 3.1-mile run.) This year I did a seven race series and I was the champion in the men's XL division!

"I know it can be hard to decide on a coach or what plan to follow; so let me tell you what else happened this year. I cannot tell you how many athletes come up to me after races and tell me what a great job I did. I had one athlete tell me that he saw me at the beginning of the year. He stated, 'If I could do these races, so could he!' He just raced his first duathlon. I also had another athlete tell me that she tried to catch me on the bike, but could not. She complimented me on my riding strength. When you gain the respect of your fellow athletes, it is worth more than any award.

"Thank you, Rick. Without your easy-to-follow nutrition and fitness program, I would have never been able to gain the respect of my fellow athletes!"

Frank Spano

"I was advised by a friend to look up Rick's Web site because he was so 'marketable'. I knew Rick was a great athlete, but I had no idea he was a nutrition and fitness coach too. After reading through the Web site, my eyes instantly got big because I knew Rick was just what I had been looking for.

"I wanted to lose weight for a long time. I could no longer eat whatever I wanted like I could when I was in my twenties. After a phone consult with Rick, he told me pretend like we never spoke and write down everything I eat for a week. This made me laugh because I was on my way to a Super Bowl party.

"I wrote down everything I ate for one week. Although Rick was not at the Super Bowl party with me, he said from reading my food diary he could see my every move at the party…three chicken wings, a handful of M&M's, seven layer dip, a couple cubes of cheese, and the list goes on and on.

"That day was a challenge. But my job at the time was an even bigger one. I worked at a deli with the biggest and best 5 oz chocolate chip cookies I've ever had. I enjoyed having one, two, sometimes three of those a day. This does not include the cookie dough I would eat while preparing them. I really had a challenge in front of me and was very scared to begin with Rick. I did not know if I would be able to stick with the daily food plan Rick had helped me put together for the following week.

"I never thought I would be afraid of food in my life, and tomorrow I had to go to work and face the fear of eating the right foods. I remember as clear as day getting through the first meal and going 'OK I did it, now when do I get to eat again?' Not for three hours. This is where I made it fun. I began to look forward to the next snack or meal because I got to eat my same yummy breakfast again if I wanted, or I could move on to a snack or lunch.

"The cookies, muffins, and all the other goodies the deli served were hard to resist. I found that if I never put a piece of the bad food in my mouth, then I was usually able to stay under control until I got to eat again. So, I chewed gum to keep my mind occupied and waited for the next several hours to pass.

"After a couple weeks it was getting easier and I had begun to fall into a nice eating routine. Sure I wanted to cheat and eat bad foods, but I reminded myself how good it felt to get on that scale and see my weight go lower each week.

"The change did not happen overnight. In fact it took almost three weeks before I began to see a drop in weight. Every week I would say to Rick, 'Am I going to get skinny?' He always help put things in perspective by saying that I did not gain the extra weight I had put on in three weeks, so why would I think I could lose all my weight in just a few weeks. He had a great point. It probably took me almost two years to get up to the 150 I now weigh, and I was thinking I would be back there in just weeks. After I looked at it like that,

I stopped asking the skinny question so much and just continued to follow Rick's plan.

"Not only did Rick make a change in my diet, but he also changed the way I worked out. When I hired Rick I was only three months away from racing in the Triathlon World Championships in Madeira Island, Portugal. I worked out all the time, but as you can see from my weight (150 pounds), it didn't matter how much I worked out if I ate anything I wanted. I always had people saying to me, 'Oh, you work out so you can eat whatever you want.' That is so wrong. To me, working out equaled a reward of food. I thought as long as you worked out you could go home and eat anything you wanted, good or bad. Rick helped me understand the importance of eating before, during, and immediately after my workouts.

"I used to think if I ate an energy bar during a bike ride, I would be putting on more weight. What I didn't understand was that I needed that energy bar or gel to help continue to burn calories. Thanks to Rick I lost fourteen pounds and have run the fastest 5Ks and 10Ks of my life. I did not get faster by going out and doing all this speed work at the track like most athletes are told to do if they want to improve their times. What Rick did was slow me down to make me fast. Yes, this is an oxymoron, but still very true. Before I began training with Rick, almost every workout I did I was anaerobic (intense). It did not matter if I was swimming, biking, ice speed skating, or running. I pushed it to the limit every workout. I thought by going as hard as possible that I would get faster and lose more weight. The exact opposite was true because by working out hard every time, my body bypassed burning fat and only burned carbohydrates. I was constantly getting injured and my body weight was not moving in the right direction.

"Rick told me to invest in a heart rate monitor. What he didn't know is I already had one, but was not sure what to do with it. I learned to do all my workouts by following the heart rate he prescribed for me. Some of my runs were so slow I felt like I was walking. He continued to encourage me and to trust the training plan. Eventually my runs at the same heart rate would get faster. I couldn't believe it when it did happen. I was now running the fastest times of my life, even faster than my high school cross-country personal records. Now those same runs are much faster, and it's all because I listened and believed in my coach.

"Thanks to Rick I will never have to buy another one of those fad diet books because he showed me a plan that I will use for the rest of my life!"

Loren Uscilowski

"My name is Nick Spano. I am fifty-three years old and will be married twenty-five years on December 22, 2004. While raising two fine sons, it was easy to neglect myself. They are now twenty-three and on their own. So it's about time that I started doing something to get myself back in shape.

"I saw Rick Kattouf in November of 2004. He set up a meeting with me on November 17. We discussed his plans for nutrition and exercise. He also told me how there is no diet involved, but rather a plan to change my eating habits for the rest of my life. His catch…it would be easy! Sure, I had heard that before. But I trusted Rick. After all, he had been a high school student of mine. And I figured that he must really know something since he is the number one duathlete in his age group in the United States.

"When he discussed the meal plan, I got excited. Eating five meals a day would be just fine for me, especially since I have been a diabetic for twenty-three years. I thought it was under control with the medication I had been taking. Rick encouraged me to review the daily log I had kept on my sugar readings and weight. I was shocked! My readings were much higher than I had thought. I had been "fooling" myself for many years.

"I went back and reviewed my stats. Some days I had good readings, but on most days they were bad. I would make notes to justify those results, like 'wedding reception' or 'holiday'. My average *almost daily* sugar readings from September of '04 until the day I started on his plan were 140, 136, 119, 121, 161, 137, 140, 133, 154, 160, and 132. It was like a roller coaster. After just three weeks on Rick's exercise and eating plan, I cannot believe the results: 103, 109, and 95!

"My weight is also staring to drop. I can't wait to see the new me! I am convinced that Dr. Rick Kattouf has the best exercise and meal plan in existence for most people. I have not had a difficult time at all for the three weeks I have been on this plan. I am eating very good meals and have even eaten out several times. You just have to 'eat smart'. Try it for yourself. If you have a difficult time believing my results, don't feel bad. I would be skeptical of claims like these, too. I will swear that the facts I have stated are true and would gladly show you my daily log sheets upon request."

Nicholas J. Spano

Appendix A

Product ordering information: Visit **www.TeamKattouf.com**, click on sponsors to link to each product site.

Baker's Breakfast Cookie:
You can order online at **www.bbcookies.com** or call 877-889-1090. Mention promotion code KAT to receive $2 off your order.

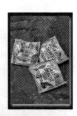

Champion Nutrition:
You can order online at **www. champion-nutrition.com** or call 800-225-4831.

MaxiVision and MaxiFlex:
You can order online at **www.medicalophthalmics.com** or call 888-290-6924. Mention promotion code KAT to receive $2 off your order.

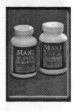

Power PB:
You can order online at **www.powerpb.com** or call 866-732-6885. Mention promotion code KAT to receive 10 percent off your order.

Go Fast:
You can order online at **www.gofastsports.com** or call 800-895-7290. Mention promotion code KAT and receive 10 percent off your order.

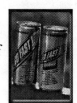

Penta water:
You can order online at **www.pentawater.com** or call 800-531-5088

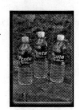

PowerCranks:
You can visit **www.powercranks.com** for product information. To order, e-mail me at **rick@rickkattouf.com,** mention promotion code KAT, and receive 10 percent off your order.

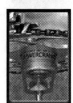

Rudy Project Eyewear:
You can order on line at **www.rx-spex.com** or call 888-950-SPEX, Mention promotion code KAT and receive a complimentary Rudy Project promotional item.

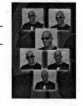

About the Author

Rick Kattouf, Nutrition and Fitness Coach, ACSM Certified Personal Trainer, and Doctor of Optometry, was born on March 22, 1971, in Oak Park, Illinois. His family moved to Warren, Ohio, in May of 1972 where his father started his optometric practice. In 1989, Rick graduated from John F. Kennedy high school in Warren. During his high school career, Rick competed in football (he received the Ann Jewel Memorial for his tireless work ethic), track (he received the "coaches award" his senior year), and basketball while graduating with a 3.5 GPA.

In August 1989, Rick enrolled in Oberlin College in Oberlin, Ohio, where he was the starting quarterback and ran track. In January 1991, Rick transferred to Kent State University in Kent, Ohio. It was at Kent State that that Rick started his nutrition and fitness coaching business. In August 1993, Rick received his premed Bachelor of Science in Zoology.

Rick entered the Illinois College of Optometry (ICO) in August 1993. This was the same optometry school that his sister Valerie (1995 ICO graduate) and his father (1972 ICO graduate) attended. During his third year of optometry school, Rick ran his first marathon in 1996. In May 1997, Rick received his Doctor of Optometry (OD) degree and his Bachelor of Science in Visual Science. At graduation, Rick was voted by the optometric faculty as "most likely to succeed" and also received the Kenneth P. Martin Alumnus of the Year award. Three days after graduation, he joined his father's optometric practice in Warren, Ohio.

The summer following graduation in 1997, he raced his first triathlon. Rick began racing duathlons in 1999. In October 2000, he raced his first duathlon world championship in Calais, France. Following the 2000 world championships, he was honored by the mayor of Warren for his accomplishments, both professionally and athletically. In June 2001, Rick gave the commencement address to the middle school in which he attended. He went on to compete in the world championships in 2001 (Rimini, Italy), 2002 (Alpharetta, Georgia), and 2003 (Alfoltern, Switzerland). In 2004, Rick was injured following a cycling accident, causing him to miss the world championships in Fredrica, Denmark. He qualified for the duathlon long course world championships in Barcis, Italy, which will take place in May 2005. At the beginning of 2003, Rick renamed his nutrition and fitness coaching business to TeamKattouf, Inc.

One very interesting aspect of Rick's athletic life has been his altitude room. He sleeps in a bedroom that simulates altitude up to 15,000 feet above sea level. He is sponsored by Colorado Altitude Training (CAT) www. altitudetraining.com. The science behind the room is to "sleep high (at altitude), train low (at sea level)." Sleeping at altitude creates an increase in red blood cell production, which improves his endurance.

Rick divides his time between northeast Ohio in Warren and southwest Florida in Bonita Springs. He is a three time all-American duathlete, *Inside Triathlon* magazine all-American duathlete. He entered the 2004 duathlon season as the #1 ranked duathlete in the USA (age 30–34) and #4 overall in the USA. Each year, Rick is invited to speak to numerous groups on nutrition and fitness. If you are interested in having Rick put on a dynamic nutrition and fitness clinic, please contact him at rick@rickkattouf.com or call 330-219-5095.

Index

978-0-595-33945-7
0-595-33945-X

CPSIA information can be obtained at www.ICGtesting.com
224340LV00001B/4/A